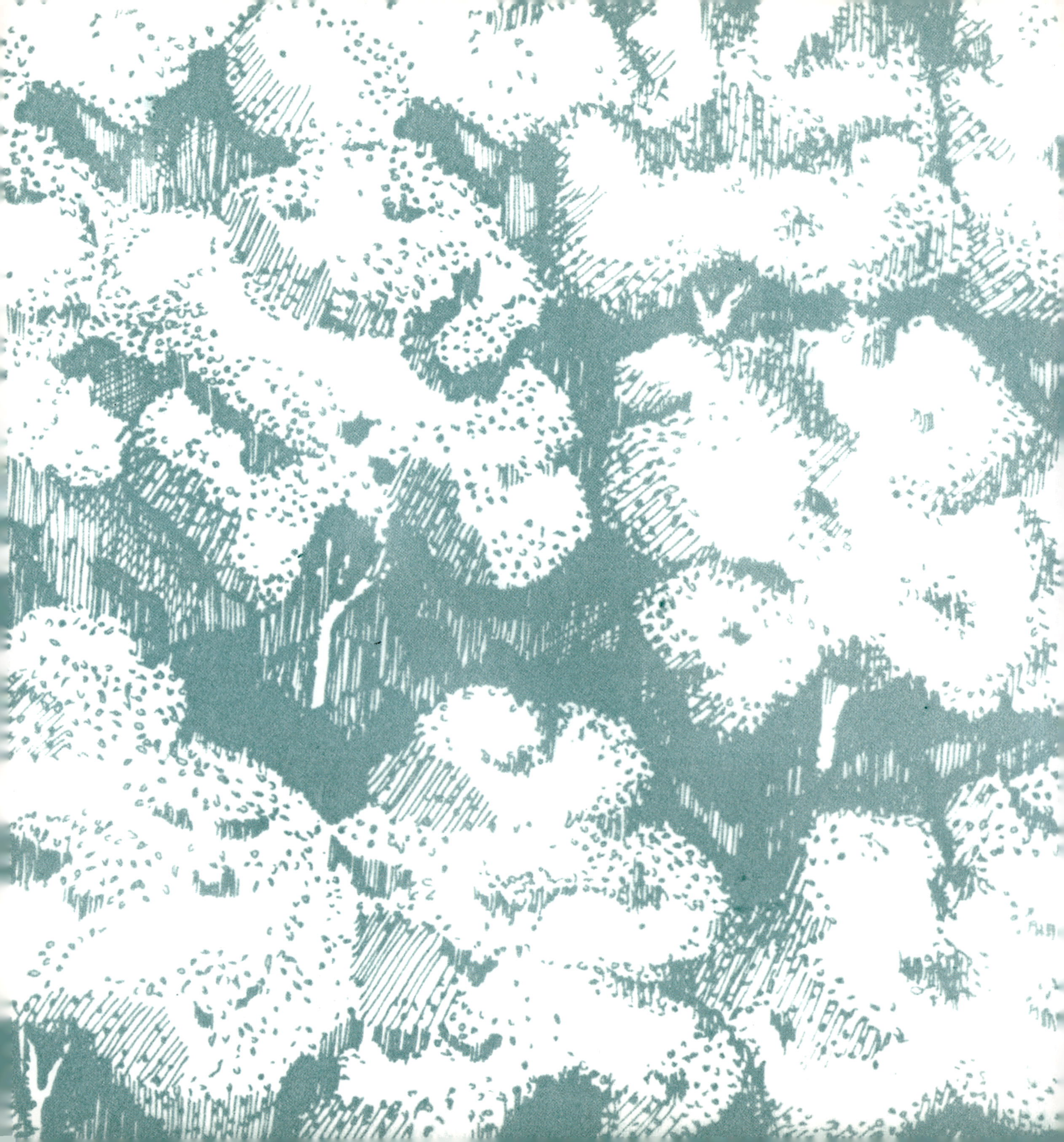

BUDDHIST HEALING IN LAOS

Best wishes

Denise Tomecko

BY THE SAME AUTHOR

Sukuma: Vanishing Tribes of Africa
Private publication 1974.

Shiva: Lord Shiva and his Yogis – co-authored with Paula Fouce
Orchid Press, Bangkok, 1990, 1996.

BUDDHIST HEALING IN LAOS

Plants of the Fragrant Forest

Denise Tomecko

Orchid Press

Denise Tomecko
BUDDHIST HEALING IN LAOS: Plants of the Fragrant Forest

ORCHID PRESS
P.O. Box 19,
Yuttitham Post Office,
Bangkok 10907 Thailand
www.orchidbooks.com

Printed in Singapore

ISBN-10: 974-524-078-8
ISBN-13: 978-974-524-078-0

Dedication

Buddhist Healing in Laos was inspired by the work of Mae-khaao Keo, Lao Buddhist nun, renowned healer and experienced meditation teacher, whose simple living and high thinking is a true inspiration in an increasingly materialistic world.

Mae-khaao Keo is a "living treasure" in the ancient art of Lao herbal lore and is responsible for running medicinal steam baths, with their accompanying treatments, both within monastery grounds and in other locations.

She is deeply concerned that the natural environment, from which so many of the medicinal plants are harvested, may soon be destroyed. She has difficulty finding dedicated apprentices to whom she can pass on her vast empirical knowledge, which requires years of study, as well as discipline in meditation.

As people move away from traditional values and local medicines in favor of modern alternatives, this precious wisdom could be lost to future generations. It was at her request that I began to record the aromatic plants prescribed at her Lao sauna, with their therapeutic benefits. This book has grown out of her request and it is my hope that any proceeds will be used to build more healing saunas in Laos, especially in areas where there is little access to modern medicine.

Mae-khaao Keo

This book is for you with deepest gratitude and affection

ACKNOWLEDGEMENTS

I would like to express my heartfelt gratitude to all the people who have contributed to this work.

A special mention must go to:

Mae-khaao Keo and Ven. Achaan Sali Khantasali, without whom this project would never have been born.

Dr J.E. Vidal, a leading expert on the flora of mainland South East Asia, for introducing me to the Lao botanist Dr Bouakaykhone Svengsuka. Thank you for your kindness and encouragement to complete this project.

Dr Bouakaykhone Svengsuka works at the National University of Laos. She gave generously of her time, and her extensive knowledge of Lao flora, to correct and complete the botanical section. Your work was completely indispensable!

Dean James Gustav Speth, School of Forestry and Environmental Studies at Yale University, USA, for providing a thought-provoking foreword to this book.

Rachel Dechainaux (Mukda), a dear friend, fellow Aromatherapy enthusiast and gifted naturalist, who has been active in helping me from the start, both as a patient Lao/English translator and plant expert in her own right. Your gentle nature and positive input have been quite invaluable, both to the process and to me personally.

Mr Nick Enfield, an expert in linguistics, who produced Lao phonetics for all the plant names and helped us overcome other errors in the text. Many thanks.

My husband Jim Tomecko, critic, editor and loyal supporter, "You are the wind beneath my wings".

Without all of you this book would never have been completed!

Thanks must also go to Mr Thongped Sanpasert (Ped) and Ms PaPhavady Keomevangsens (Noi), from the Wat Sok Paa Luang sauna for their explanations of daily sauna work.

And to my long suffering friends:

Hermene Rodenburg, my Dharma sister, who believed in me all along and made me think that I could do it when I lost hope. Thanks for being there.

Nuan Chan, my Lao companion, for introducing me to helpful Buddhist contacts and assisting with translations. You brought me to the heart of your culture with openness and joy. You touched my life.

Japo Khen, who inspired me with his purity, simplicity and focus on the Buddhist path.

Michele and Peter Horn who did so much

to help organise the artwork for this book. I am very grateful.

Ashli Varma, new friend and journalist, for giving me some very useful suggestions and editing the work.

Andrew Ingles, for the valuable input on ecological matters. You spoke to me of Lao and the practical things that could be done there, and elsewhere, to save our natural world.

Margaret Ingles, a true and honest friend, who has a special place in my heart. Thanks for your encouragment

The long process of completing this work has been a personal journey as well as a literary one. I have learned much about the generosity of the human spirit, about the diversity of Buddhist life in South East Asia and have been honoured to enter the lives and work of some of its people.

If others benefit from this book it is as a direct result of the guidance of my precious teachers and the patient kindness of my friends. If it contains mistakes or misconceptions, they are purely a result of my own shortcomings, and if they are too numerous—I apologise.

"If you can find a friend to go with you, who is steady, careful and mature, together you can overcome all hardships with mindfulness and joy."

Dharmapada – PG 163

CONTENTS

LIST OF ILLUSTRATIONS

The beautiful watercolours in this book were created in Laos by two talented Lao artists, Mr Sackda Bophoamphalack and Mr Tingkham Sengaphay. In the list of illustrations below, their initials indicate which of the paintings are the work of each artist. In addition, Mr Sackda Bophoamphalack kindly provided the small details used as chapter decorations.

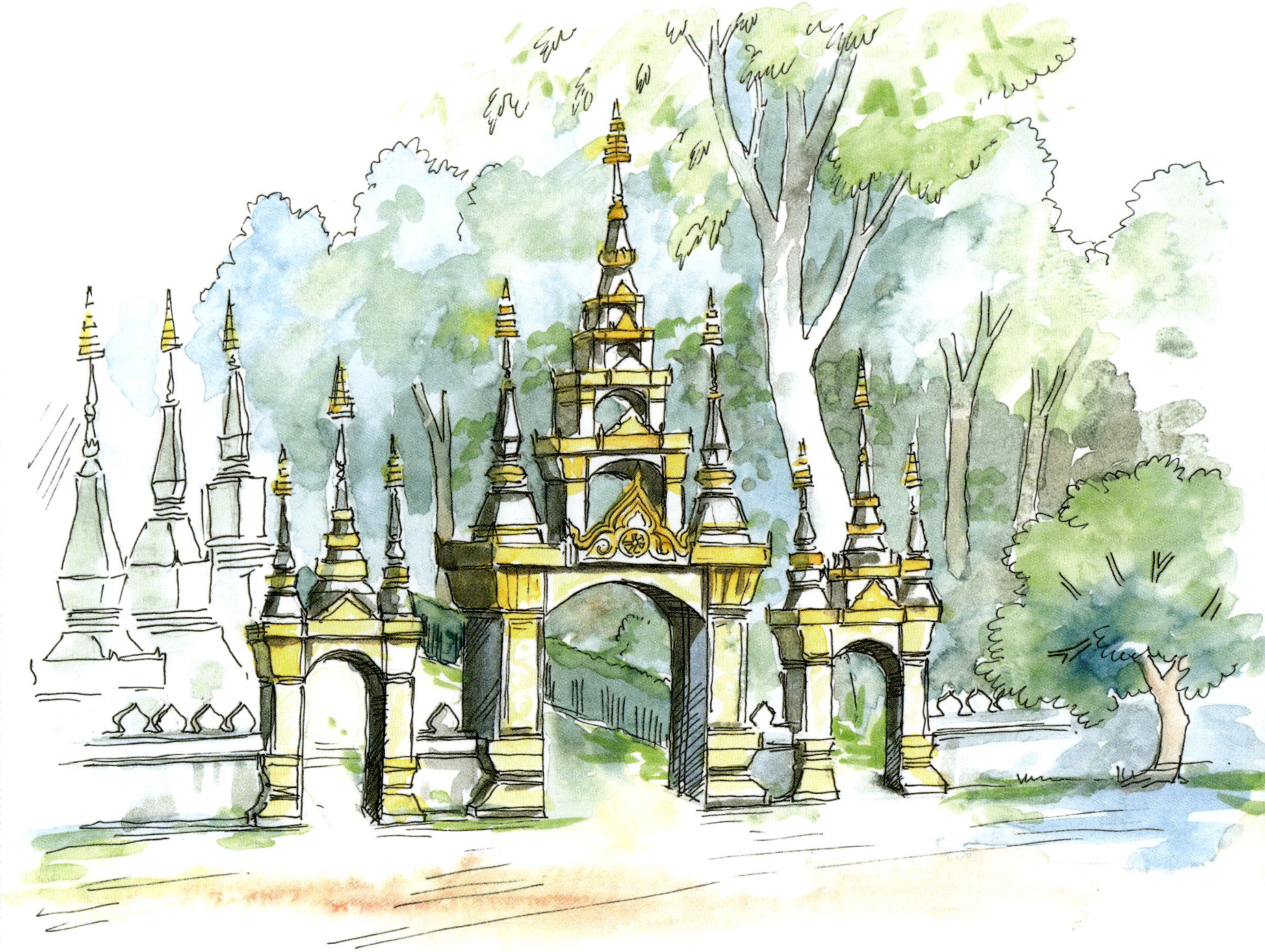

FOREWORD

The Heart of the Matter

When people ask me today, "What is the most important issue in the world?" I reply "It's the business of bringing our human enterprise into harmony with the natural world, a world of which we are just a part." I think the truth of this statement will become clear in the years ahead. The enormous expansion of the human enterprise in recent years has brought us to the threshold of a fundamentally new era, an era in which our ability to manage the environment must quickly emerge as the top priority of governments and to people everywhere. Denise Tomecko's book highlights what can be achieved in a healthy environment, where human need rather than human greed, has precedence, and where human endeavor, medicine and optimization of the natural world have found harmonious balance—at least for a time. This is certainly not true for much of the world.

Consider first what has already happened. Half of the world's tropical and temperate forests are gone. About half of the wetlands and a third of the mangrove are also gone. Ninety percent of the large predator fish are gone, and seventy-five percent of marine fisheries are now over fished or fished to capacity. Twenty percent of the corals are gone and another twenty percent severely threatened. Species are disappearing at rates of a 100 to a 1,000 times faster than normal. Most agricultural land in drier regions suffers from serious deterioration. Persistent toxic chemicals can now by found, by the dozens, in each and every one of us. Environmental losses are already great!

Still, we continue to push atmospheric carbon dioxide up, starting the dangerous process of warming the planet and disrupting its climate. Everywhere the earth's ice fields are melting. We already consume or destroy each year about 40% of nature's photosynthetic output, crowding out other species. Our demands on water mean that some of the world's mightiest of rivers such as the Ganges, Yellow, Nile and Colorado no longer reach the oceans in the dry season. Will the Mekong be the next victim of human manipulation?

And one of the more sobering facts is that our thirst for economic growth is pushing us further and faster in the same direction. The world's economy is poised to double and then double again by the middle of this century. Somehow this economic growth cannot resemble the growth of the past; it requires new designs and new technologies. Everything must be different—construction, manufacturing, energy production, transportation, forestry and agriculture—all very different. Only unprecedented action taken with a profound sense of urgency can forestall an appalling deterioration of our natural assets. This is the challenge of "environmental management".

It is fortunate that we are now in the midst of a paradigm shift in our thinking about environmental management. In earlier times the environmental style was confrontational, business was the enemy. Today we put collaboration ahead of confrontation; rather than putting polluters in straight jackets we try to use the incentives and disincentives of market mechanisms to develop the technologies to get us out of this mess. Now we recognize that the market can be guided for environmental as well as economic goals. And that guidance requires government action to get the prices right—environmentally honest prices.

Where we used to concentrate on environmental protection, now we realize that if we do not include the development of poorer countries in our scheme of things, we can never sustain the earth's biosphere. This has led us into the art and science of sustainable development, where the aim is to achieve success in economics, the environment and society at the same time.

While we may look to the government for leadership, we also know that business is often ahead of government; scientists are often ahead of government; consumers and environmentalists are often ahead of government. We cannot always wait for government; we have to push forward in the knowledge that while politicians ride the waves, it is the citizens that make the waves. It is this affirmation of action that Wallace Stevens refers to in his writings when he says "After the final no there comes a yes and on that yes the future of the world depends." Despite the deeply daunting projections of environmental decline, we affirm that we will win this struggle for the future and that the forests that are the source of Lao traditional medicine will still be with us as we embark on the next century.

James Gustave Speth
Dean, School of Forestry
and Environmental Studies
Yale University

A SHORT HISTORY OF LAOS

Due to its location in the centre of the South East Asian peninsula, Laos has been at a crossroads of culture and trade for hundreds of years.

The area we now call Laos was until the 14th century a collection of small states that had, at various times in the 11th and 12th centuries been annexed by the Khmers and Mons (not Thais—they were not here then). In 1353, a Lao prince named Fan Ngum, assumed the throne of Luang Prabang in what is now northern Laos. He united many of the small states and founded his own kingdom, which he called Lan Xang or the Land of a Million Elephants. He established Theravada Buddhism as the state religion.

After 1707 however, dynastic feuds once more divided the country, this time into three main competing kingdoms: Luang Prabang, the traditional seat of power in the north; Vientiane in the centre; and Champasak in the south, as well as smaller city states such as Xieng Khouang and Muang Sing.

By the 19th century Thailand was trying to annex the divided Laos and this was only averted by Laos' direct appeal for protection to the French colonial powers that had governed Indochina for more than a hundred years. After France accepted this request, Laos became a French protectorate and was reunited once more under the royal house of Luang Prabang. During this time it was left relatively unexploited by its French protectors largely because of its impenetrable forests, its small and sparsely dispersed population and limited navigational opportunities along the Mekong River. The country remained a protectorate of French Indochina until World War II when it came under Japanese occupation. However, with the final defeat of Japan at the end of the war, King Sisavang Vong of Luang Prabang accepted the reestablishment of French control in exchange for continued protection during a period of political uncertainty when political boundaries were particularly vulnerable. This return of control to the French was strongly opposed by the Free Lao, an anti-French movement, which had formed a government in exile in neighboring Thailand. Therefore, even though Laos later joined the French Union as a semi-autonomous state and in 1953 was granted full independence, the Free Lao movement had already evolved into a communist backed revolutionary group known as the Pathet Lao which had managed to establish control over many areas in the north of the country.

A prolonged and bloody civil war ensued between the communist Pathet Lao and the Royal Government of Laos. It was not until 1974 that a coalition government was formed between the opposing sides. But this did not last long because, while all this infighting was going on, the Vietnam War was increasingly affecting the politics of Laos. While the Americans secretly supported the Royalists in exchange for air space and permission to run secret missions through the country from Thailand into Vietnam, the Vietnamese communists were sustaining the Pathet Lao. Soon after the fall of South Vietnam and Cambodia to the Communists in 1975, the Pathet Lao managed to assume full control of the country. The party changed the country's name to the Lao Peoples Democratic Republic, or Lao PDR, and the monarchy was abolished. Thereafter for almost twenty years the country closed its doors on the west and embraced one party state communism.

The communist takeover was followed by a time of persecution for many former officials and supporters of the royal government. Some were sent to the infamous "re-education camps", while hundreds of thousands of others left the country as refugees, including most of the educated elite and many Buddhist monks and nuns. Buddhist teachings in schools were forbidden and lay people were not permitted to gain merit by feeding the monks. Monks were obligated to do physical work each day and were not permitted to meditate or chant. They could however, at the request of the people, perform social services such as presiding at funerals and other secular activities. Because of these services, the temples were left largely intact.

Just two years after the communist takeover, Laos signed a treaty of peace and friendship with Vietnam initiating a period during which Vietnam agreed to provide Laos with aid to develop its agriculture, forestry, industries, and transportation. They also gave Laos duty-free access to the seaport facilities at Da Nang as well as substantial military support. The alliance with Vietnam expanded to include the Soviet Block after Vietnam invaded Cambodia in 1979. As these relationships matured over the next ten years self-reliance was stressed in all areas of life including that of medicine. The Lao Government encouraged the use of locally available medicines in the place of more "western" methods, which, in any case were unaffordable. They conducted scientific research into the uses and chemical constituents of traditional medicines resulting in an active revival of the traditional medicine that has continued until today.

In 1989, with the collapse of Soviet style Marxism in Eastern Europe, the Lao leadership was forced to seek more economic aid and investment from the West by professing a more liberal economic orientation to "state capitalism". To reassure western governments and foreign investors, they reduced obvious connections with the Vietnamese military, normalized relations with China and produced a government development plan. The plan called for investments in infrastructure, privatization of state enterprises, rural development and reforms in health services and education. Laos continues to receive foreign aid and is developing quickly.

THE AUTHOR'S STORY

I did not know what to expect. Like most people, I associated Laos with memories of the Vietnam War, jungles and guerrilla warfare—a mysterious place largely unknown to the outside world. As the plane circled the runway, I recall looking down on a startlingly green landscape composed of a lush network of rice cultivation, forest and jungle; in the distance an outline of grey hills merged with the sky. Weaving its way through this sea of green was a brown serpentine river, the mighty Mekong, rising in Tibet and making its way through China, Burma, Laos, Thailand and Cambodia to the sea. All along its banks shone the sparkling roofs of Buddhist temples, their highly glazed tiles shimmering like gold in the sun.

Vientiane, with its wide tree-lined roads and its blend of French colonial, modern and traditional Lao architecture, appeared more like a charming country town than the capital city. The generous use of teak and rosewoods in Lao homes is stunning to the Western eye. The oldest houses are completely constructed of teak with beautifully carved details, large airy rooms and porches. They stand on stilts to avoid the monsoon rains and rising rivers.

Vientiane became our home for the next five years and a precious chapter in the story of our lives. As my husband settled into his new job involved with the development of small private sector businesses, I was not sure what opportunities were in store for me. So, I decided to leave myself open and simply absorb the new environment.

The lifestyle in Vientiane was very easy going, or "sabai, sabai" as they say locally. In the beginning I found it so slow that I thought I would simply fall into an eternal slumber. But, as I became accustomed to the tempo of daily life I was soon seduced by the slow pace and the friendliness of the people.

As in many hot countries, it is common for people to take a siesta in the afternoon preferring, as they do, to work in the earlier and later hours of the day when the sun is less intense. In the cool of the evening the town's street cafes and restaurants, particularly along the banks of the Mekong, came to life with groups of friends catching up with the day's news, taking great pleasure in the sharing of food and beer. This is not considered a luxury or special treat, but an essential part of everyday life. Their ability to have fun together in this simple way, day after day, caused me to consider how much we have lost in the West with our overly busy lives.

In the early nineties, when we arrived, the age of TV and computers had not yet been sufficiently established to change these time-honoured customs. In fact the communist government had just banned the use of the Internet when we arrived in Laos, and phones were still occasionally tapped. The few people who could afford a TV watched Thai programs, which they could pick up from broadcasting stations just across the border over the Mekong. Lao TV consisted mainly of state controlled news, and was obviously not as popular as a good Thai 'soap'. The north-eastern Thai and the Lao culture have a lot in common and at certain times in the history of the country, Lao territories extended far into what is now northern Thailand.

After we had found ourselves a house to rent, I set about exploring my new neighbourhood. It was also around this time that I met Nuan, my first Lao friend. She was to become an early guide, patient translator and cultural advisor. One hot Sunday morning I took a walk, with Nuan, to our local Buddhist Temple or Wat, just for a quick look and perhaps to meet some of the monks and nuns. As a Buddhist family, this seemed like a nice way for us to connect with our neighbours. I did not know it at that time but our local Wat, called Sok Paa Luang, was one of the more important monasteries in the country.

We arrived at a large, impressive looking gate on the road (see p. xii), beyond which lay what appeared to be a forest. From the gate we could not see any buildings, just trees and shrubs, with a dirt road leading into the grounds. A timeless sense of peace and quiet exuded from the place. As we wandered down the road, we soon began to see tiny wooden houses built on stilts, dotted amongst the foliage. These were the living quarters and meditation huts of the monks and nuns. I remember thinking how different it all was from the grand, richly decorated Tibetan monasteries that I was used to, after living for more than seven years in Nepal. What a contrast this place was, its simplicity at once quietened the mind and washed away physical tensions. I was impressed!

Nuan took me to meet the Abbot, Ven. Achaan Sali Khantasali, and translated on my behalf. The Ven. Achaan could not have been more welcoming and asked us many questions about our family and how we came to be living in Laos. He seemed eager to talk about world events and the spread of Buddhism in the West, which he found of particular interest. We stayed for a long time, chatting away like old friends. He told us to consider Wat Sok Paa Luang our family temple and that we would always be welcome there. We came away feeling as if we had found a new spiritual friend and a gifted Buddhist teacher. I did not realise then just how special he was, or how connected we would become over the following years.

The forest around the monastery covered quite a large area and, as we wandered around, I noticed the fragrance of aromatic plants in the air. This became stronger as we approached an old Lao styled wooden building on stilts. It was a traditional herbal steam bath and the focal point of a healing centre run by the Wat's nuns. I was later told by a Lao friend that the presence of many nuns in a temple is sure sign of the availability of really good Buddhist teaching and practise. The reason for this is interesting. Since nuns have little or no chance of rising in the male dominated religious hierarchy of a monastery, they tend to gather in places where they can get high quality Buddhist teachings and fair treatment. In Sok Paa Luang the nuns not only served the monks, as one finds in most Wats, but they also had a genuine opportunity to study, meditate and even teach. Ven. Achaan Sali's profound teachings, and the fair treatment they received, attracted many sincere seekers both male and female.

During our tour we met one particular nun, who impressed me very much. Her name was Mae-khaao Keo, a tiny woman with incredible vitality, radiance and bright, twinkling eyes. We found her busily tending her garden of medicinal plants but as we approached she was happy to stop and talk with us. She was in charge of the herbal healing centre and was a fund of information on Lao curative plants and their uses. It was common, she explained, for people to come for regular steam baths on their way home from work, or on the weekends, for the improvement of their health and the prevention of disease. She also treated patients with specific illnesses by prescribing selective plants for the steam room. She also gave people advice and spiritual guidance in times of trouble. Having spent the past five years studying and practicing Aromatherapy myself, I was fascinated and overjoyed that I had stumbled on a treasure trove of traditional knowledge.

It seemed that these old medical traditions had been retained, more or less intact over the years. This was partly because of the communist government's xenophobic attitude toward the outside world and also because of a lack of hard currency to import foreign medicine. So, the healers and their patients had to fall back on their own practical knowledge of the indigenous healing plants growing in their fields and tropical forests. In fact, this turned out to be a great blessing, as similar knowledge has been lost in many other parts of the region.

Several weeks passed after these initial introductions, as I got caught up in the many details of settling into a new country and meeting people. I had not been back to the Wat. Then early one morning a messenger arrived from Sok Paa Luang to say that Ven. Achaan Sali would like to see me. I was both excited and intrigued.

After the polite preliminaries, Ven. Achaan explained the purpose of our meeting. He mentioned that an increasing number of Westerners were coming to the monastery and asking to receive Buddhist teachings. He pointed out that there had not been an opportunity in the past to teach many Westerners and wondered how he might go about organising something for them. Since I had had some experience in organising such events I offered to help and, to this end, elicited the help of another new friend, and fellow Buddhist, Hermene Rodenburg. Hermene was well versed in organising Buddhist courses and seminars in the West and was happy to be involved. Being fluent in Lao and having lived in the region for a long time she was a great asset. So, after much discussion, a date was picked and a weekend course was arranged. We were requested to advertise this only by word of mouth, since the authorities were still extremely suspicious of activities involving Westerners. We eventually spent a wonderful weekend of meditation and cultural exchange with about twenty participants.

This weekend of teaching and meditation became a bi-annual event and expanded into a regular Saturday afternoon silent meditation session that continues to this day, attracting both foreigners and Lao Buddhists. We passed many wonderful hours with our friends in the tranquillity of the monastery grounds and it became the highlight of our week. What was most attractive about those days was the totally un-commercialized atmosphere of the place and the beauty of simply "being" together in the Lao way.

During these sessions I also grew closer to Mae-khaao Keo and we began to meet regularly at the steam room. We had quiet conversations about the sauna and the plants that she used for healing; we also discussed Lao and Western approaches to Aromatherapy. She introduced me to one young nun who was trying to learn about the medicinal plants and healing methods, but due to the tough discipline and years of study required she gave up. Mae-khaao said this was not unusual and was concerned that her knowledge could be lost forever if she were not able to find a suitable apprentice. It pained me to consider that her knowledge may not be passed on or even recorded. I began to wonder if I could make a small contribution by at least documenting the sauna plants and their uses for future generations. Mae-khaao expressed her wish that I should do this and I hope this book will, in some small way, contribute to the preservation of this valuable tradition.

The main body of the work introduces the therapeutic benefits of traditional herbal saunas, and other aromatic methods used in Laos today, as well as their impact, not only on the cure of physical ailments but also on the human mind. I have listed the plants with their Lao names, botanical names, therapeutic uses and descriptions, and included water colour illustrations, for the use of prospective healers.

I hope to convince the reader that herbal and aromatic healing can truly enrich modern allopathic medicine in a complementary way, a way that could create a more integrated approach to future medicine and a way that many patients already want.

INTRODUCTION

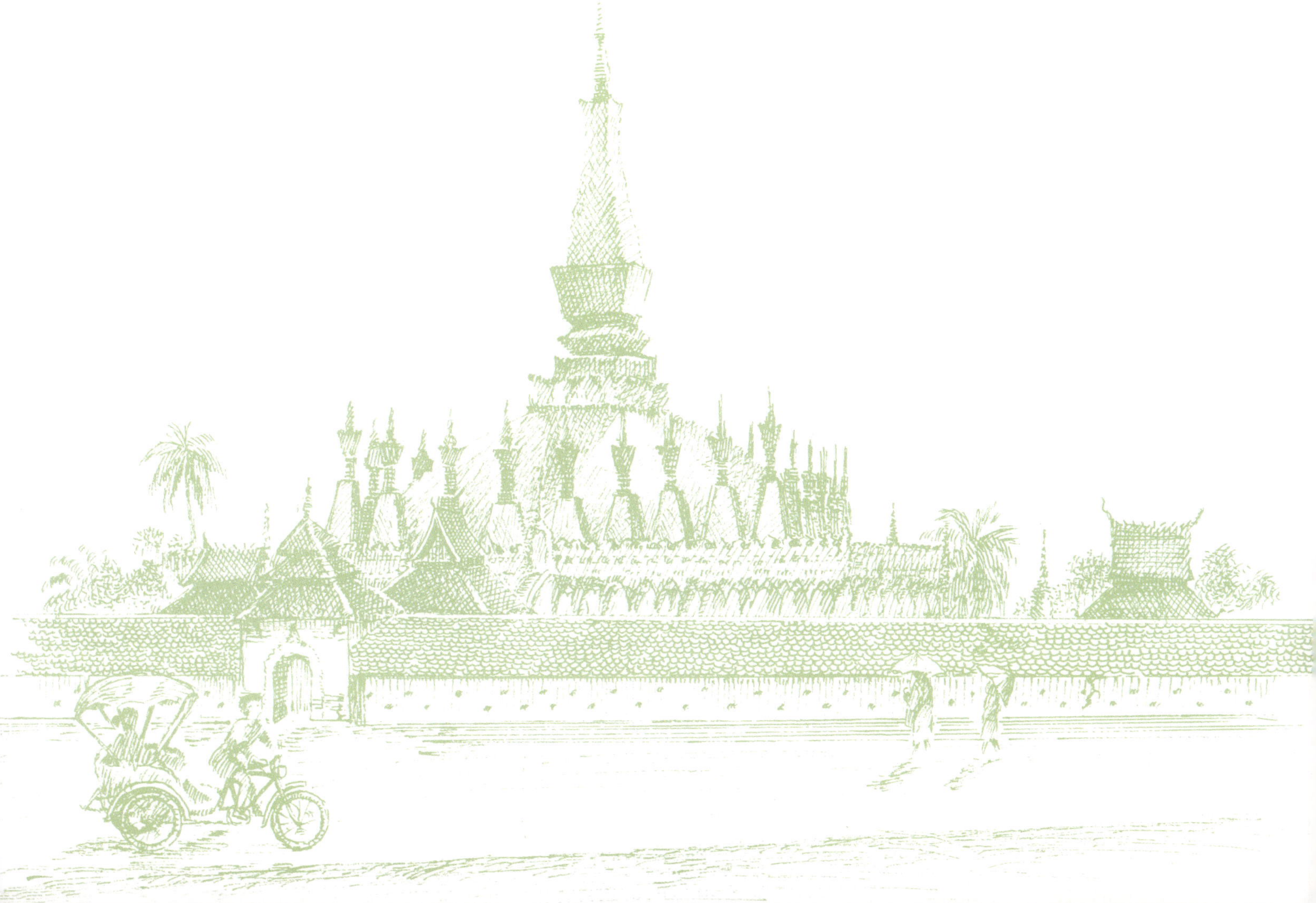

INTRODUCTION

The quest for a healthy, pain-free body and a happy, peaceful mind has played an essential role in the development of mankind from the grasslands of Africa to the great river based civilizations of Egypt, Persia, China and India. It is a quest that continues to this day, as we constantly look for new and better ways to improve our health, happiness and longevity.

Successful early humans survived because they experimented with the resources they found in their environment. By trial and error they identified edible vegetation that could be used as food, as well as poisonous varieties that had to be avoided. They came across unusual plants that induced hallucinations, soothed emotions or relieved illnesses. As society developed and people formed themselves into larger groups, certain individuals became recognized as healers and shamans. It was their responsibility to cure the sick and to ward off negative influences both from within the community and from the world outside. Over time they accumulated a great body of empirical knowledge, which was passed on orally from one generation to the next. This knowledge seemed mysterious to the uninitiated and, as often happens with the inexplicable, it became the feared and then the magical. Early healer/shamans used hallucinogenic plants, incantations, prayers, spells and rituals to intervene with the unseen world of spirits, as well as their knowledge of plant lore to heal the sick or prevent the spread of disease. This pattern of development was widespread throughout the ancient world, until the emergence of the first larger urban settlements. These more advanced societies developed writing skills and it is among their records that we find the first known treatises on medicine and religion.

One of these early town cultures appeared in what is now northern India and Pakistan. It became known as the Indus Valley civilization, since it developed on the vast alluvial plains of the Indus River and its tributaries. These ancient peoples developed a sophisticated way of life that reached its peak around 2,500 BCE. Their religious practices, which included ritual bathing, animal sacrifice and fertility rites, as well as their laws and philosophies, were to influence Indian and South Asian thinking for thousands of years.

A central part of Indian history comes from texts known as Vedas, which were probably written by the indigenous people themselves but may also have been brought to the Indus Valley by migrating Aryan tribes from Iran in around 1,500 BCE. The earliest of these texts provide valuable historical records and it was largely due to the discipline of orthodox Vedic priests, called Brahmins, that they have come down to us today more or less intact. The Brahmins memorized their knowledge by rote and passed it on orally, until the advent of written script when it was organized and recorded. This period opened the door to the emergence of reform sects such as Jainism and Buddhism. While these reform sects did retain some aspects of earlier Vedic thinking, their inspiration came mainly from the teachings of forest ascetics.

The Brahmins guarded their knowledge and their high position within the community. The priesthood was hereditary and only they were permitted to learn the sacred language and content of the Vedas. In this way they were able to keep the knowledge to themselves, forcing citizens to seek them out as the sole providers of elaborate, and often expensive, religious or social rituals that were deemed essential to either please the gods or to appease negative forces.

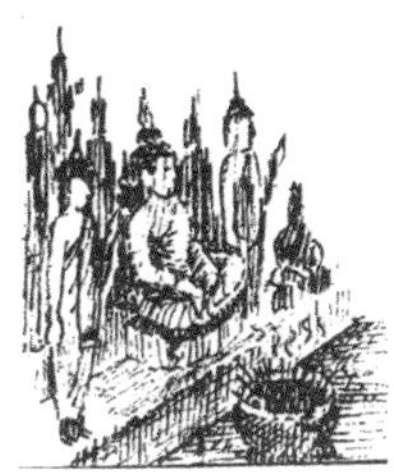

The emergence of Buddhism

Over the ensuing centuries the early settlements of the Indus Valley were replaced by a much wider network of villages and towns. As a result a gradual diversification of the society took place, which led to more independent thinking. Some people began to feel that orthodox religious beliefs, based as they were on the Vedas and the authority of the Brahmin priesthood, had become too restrictive. A trend developed towards more direct spiritual self expression with a number of young men, including Brahmins, leaving their homes to live as mendicants in the forest. There they studied with the spiritual teachers, gurus, of their day, practicing asceticism and mystical meditations. From this period of ardent spiritual exploration came a body of texts known as the Upanishads. The Upanishads are of a mystical nature, dealing with philosophical and metaphysical questions. They are best known for their doctrine positing an ultimate, universal reality of pure being and its identity with the innermost essence of the human individual. Due to its profundity, the philosophy of the Upanishads eventually became known as Vedanta or "the end of the Vedas", containing a freedom of thought unknown in earlier works.

One such forest ascetic was a young prince by the name of Siddhartha Gautama (563–483 BCE), who left his wealthy home and family to pursue his own spiritual quest in the forests of northern India. Siddhartha wandered from place to place, studying with famous teachers and practicing their different spiritual disciplines, in the hope of finding answers to the questions that troubled him; what were the real causes of suffering in the world and was there a way to lasting happiness? However after many years of diligent training, and the practice of severe austerities, his efforts did not seem to have brought him any closer to the answers he sought. Feeling that he was no longer making progress, Siddhartha went off to meditate alone and, seating himself under a sacred tree, resolved to find his answers or die in the attempt. During the course of his deep meditations, he developed profound insights into the causes of suffering, as well as a path towards genuine happiness and, at last, had a complete epiphany or enlightenment, known as Nirvana. Among the devoted followers who soon gathered around him, he became known as the Buddha or Awakened One; a young prince who had, through his own efforts, resolved some of the greatest mysteries of life. The Buddha became deeply respected, even by the orthodox schools, as one of the most celebrated teachers, thinkers and philosophers of his day. He also became an active social reformer and it was partly due to his radical new ideas that he became so influential.

He broke away from the Hindu orthodoxy and its dependence on priestly intervention with the gods, as well as its arguments relating to the existence of a single God, a pantheon of gods or to the non-existence of God altogether. Although he continued to enjoy lively debates with other teachers on the established doctrines of the time, he felt that arguments about God, which could never be proved or disproved, were not particularly useful. He stressed instead self-reliance, replacing the concept of blind faith with the possibility of a direct experience of wisdom based on study, contemplation and meditation.

He made spiritual life more accessible to the common people by teaching in their local language of Maghadi, rather than using the religious language of Sanskrit, and although he retained the Vedic theory of karma with its cycles of rebirth, he criticized fatalism as an obstacle for self-development. In particular he challenged the established caste, or class, system where a person's status at birth was fixed for the rest of their life and controversially included women in his monastic community.

The Buddha focused on a philosophy of life whose goal it was to alleviate the root causes of suffering; to cultivate a way to lasting happiness and to experience the joyful revelation of Nirvana. Nirvana was to be achieved through understanding the Four Noble Truths and practicing the Noble Eightfold Path.

The Four Noble Truths are at the core of Buddhist philosophy consisting of: the truth of suffering, the truth of the cause of suffering, the truth of the end of suffering and the truth of the path that leads to the end of suffering.

The Truth of Suffering is the recognition that suffering is an intrinsic part of life, and that it is experienced through negative emotions such as pain, dissatisfaction, discontent, unhappiness,

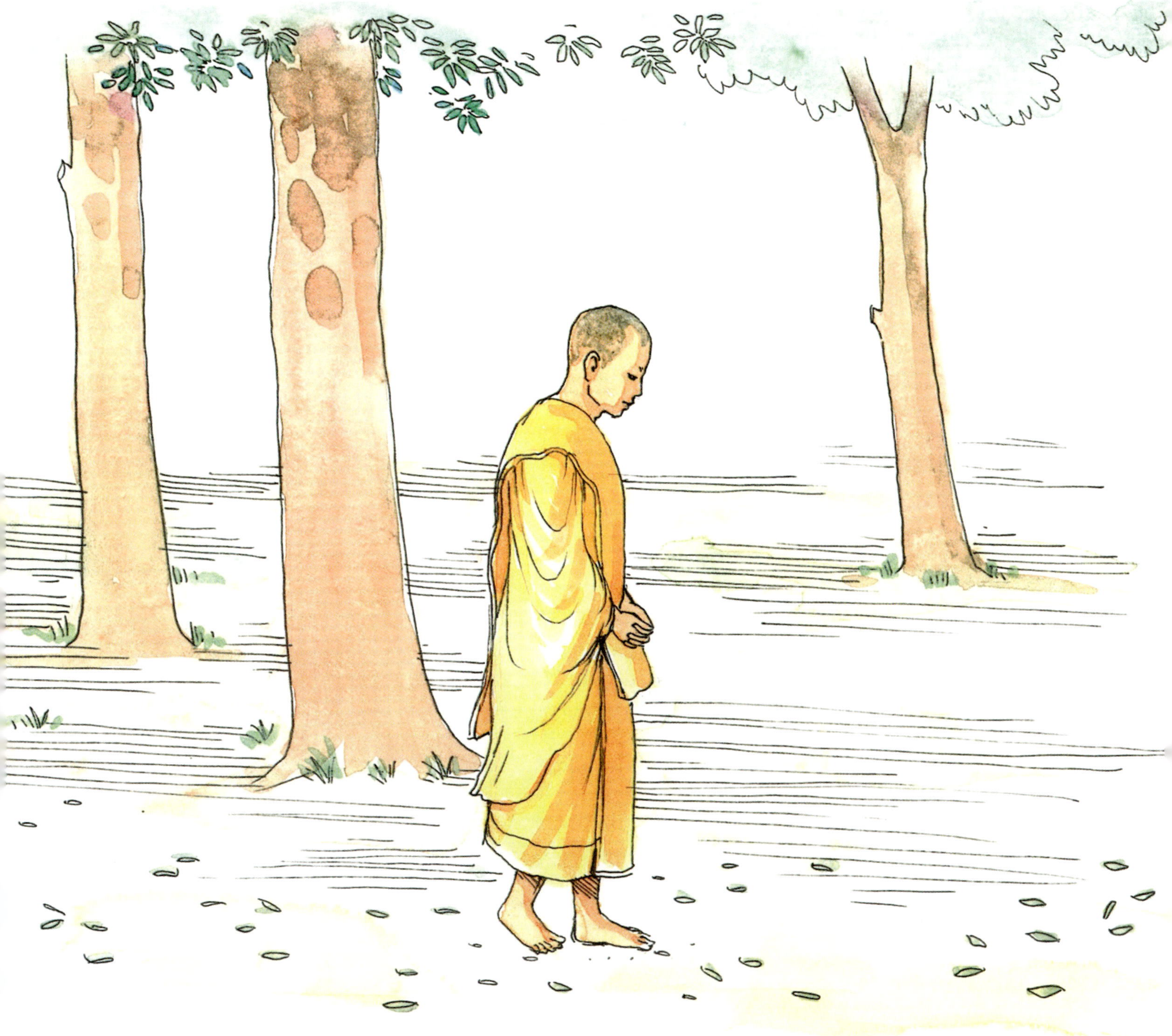

grief and impermanence.

The Truth of the Cause of Suffering is that the cause of suffering is self-centered desire and egocentricity, with all its attachments and unfullfilled expectations.

The Truth of the End of Suffering tells of a way out of suffering; a way to ease the clinging to 'me and mine' and to eliminate self-centered desires, attachments and expectations.

The Truth of the Path is a description of the way, or method, to achieve this goal. He called it "The Noble Eightfold Path", a process that promises a journey to enlightenment, through ethics, meditation and wisdom. The Noble Eightfold Path combines the practices of; right understanding, right thought, right speech, right action, right livelihood, right effort, right mindfulness and right concentration or meditation, into an integrated system of personal development.

The Four Noble Truths were often compared, by the Buddha, to four steps that had been developed in the medical sciences of ancient India. These consisted of disease, diagnosis, cure and treatment. The truth of suffering was compared to the existence of a disease; the cause of suffering to the discovery of the cause of the illness or its diagnosis; the end of suffering to identifying a suitable cure; and the path to the end of suffering to the actual treatment and cure of the illness, bringing health and happiness to the patient.

The people of Laos follow a branch of Buddhism known as the Theravada, which arrived from India via Burma, Cambodia and Sri Lanka and is now the official religion.

The Theravada or, "Doctrine of the Elders," is a school of Buddhism that draws its scriptural inspiration from a Pali canon, called the Tripitaka. Most scholars agree that the Tripitaka contains the earliest surviving record of the Buddha's teachings. The doctrines of Theravada Buddhism correspond with the basic teachings of the Buddha, including the Four Noble Truths and the idea that physical reality is based on a chain of causes and effects. Theravada Buddhism is by nature an esoteric religion, based on the practice of mediation, concentration and following the Noble Eightfold Path. It emphasizes the ideal of self-purification toward a goal of spiritual perfection known as nirvana, to be achieved through personal effort and discipline. As a result, it emphasizes monastic life, removed from the hustle and bustle of society.

Therevada is the predominant religion of Laos, Thailand, Myanmar/Burma, Cambodia and Sri Lanka. Today Theravada Buddhists number well over 100 million worldwide.

Buddhism and the origins of classical South Asian medicine

Familiarity with natural medicines was commonplace among the different groups of wandering ascetics who lived co-dependently with the forest and its environs. Some scholars have even proposed that, contrary to the popular belief that it was Brahmin intellectuals who were the main contributors to the development of Indian medicine, it was in fact based largely on the medical lore transmitted by these heterodox ascetics, particularly Buddhists. Early Buddhist monasteries were actively involved in the development of medical knowledge and it was also among the Buddhists that such knowledge first became integrated into religious doctrines and monastic disciplines. Medical references are a recurrent theme in early Buddhist texts and there is evidence to show that some monasteries ran infirmaries. These health centers may have played a significant role in the institutionalization of Indian medicine. Healing practices in Buddhist monasteries were encouraged by the Buddha himself, as can be seen in the following quote from one of his recorded sermons:

> "You, monks have neither a mother nor a father who could nurse you. If you do not nurse one another, who, then, will nurse you? Whoever would nurse me, he should nurse the sick."

Perhaps "nursing the sick" began as a necessary service to the monastic community but, with time, monk doctors treated the lay community as well. This may have served to stimulate the development of mutually reinforcing roles within the society and to guarantee support for the monasteries by the laity.

Buddhism has continued, throughout its history, to retain a connection with the healing arts. Medical courses were offered in early Buddhist universities and their medical texts were among the first of a kind. The rare manuscripts that have survived from that time are mainly practical handbooks and manuals. They list ailments and detail the herbs, or compounds, that should be administered to cure them. According to this hypothesis, the body of knowledge that ascetics, and Buddhists, had collected over the years was later included amongst the Vedic texts and called Ayurveda or "the science of life". The Ayurveda has exerted a long and pervasive effect on indigenous healing traditions throughout the Indian subcontinent as well as its neighboring regions.

The spread of Buddhism and Buddhist medicine

Even though Buddhism gained popularity in South Asia, it was not until the reign of the Indian Emperor Ashoka (232–273 BCE), who enthusiastically adopted Buddhism as the state religion, that Buddhism spread quickly to other parts of Asia. Ashoka sent missionaries along established trade routes between India, South East Asia and the Far East, via the Bay of Bengal. Over the following centuries merchants and missionaries were instrumental in bringing powerful Indian influences to mainland Southeast Asia and beyond. Buddhist missionaries traveled west to Kashmir, Pakistan, Afghanistan and even to Europe; north to Nepal; east to Burma, Thailand, Laos, Cambodia and Indonesia, while others brought the Buddhist teachings to Sri Lanka.

For the peoples of mainland South East Asia, a region that lies east of India, south of China and that is culturally influenced by both, the arrival of Buddhist monks, Hindu priests and traders from the Indian sub-continent heralded the start of a new era. While Vietnam harnessed more Chinese influences, Laos, Cambodia and Thailand were deeply affected by Indian culture, religion and medical expertise. Pharmacopoeias flourished all along the trade routes, where healing methods and remedies were traded. Eventually Laos, and other countries in the region, developed their own systems of traditional medicine based firmly on the Indian model but enriched by locally available plants and cures.

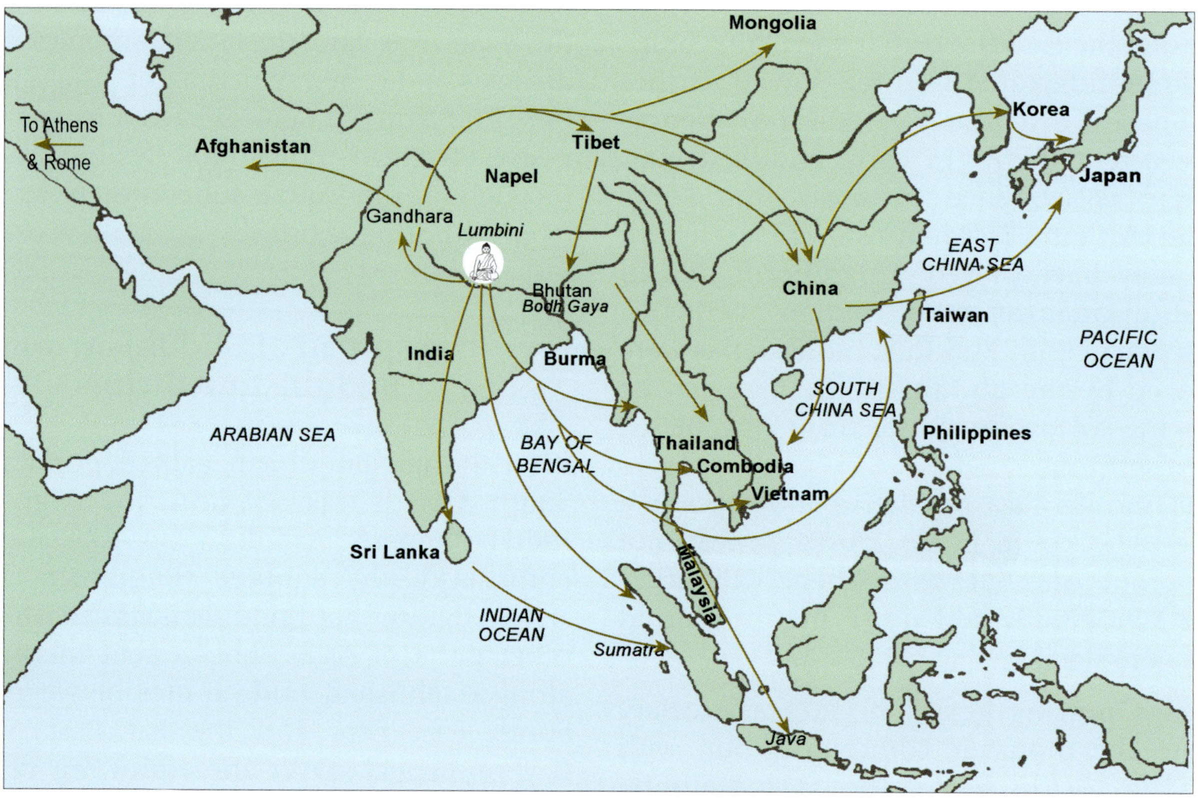

The Spread of Early Buddhism.

LAO TRADITIONAL MEDICINE

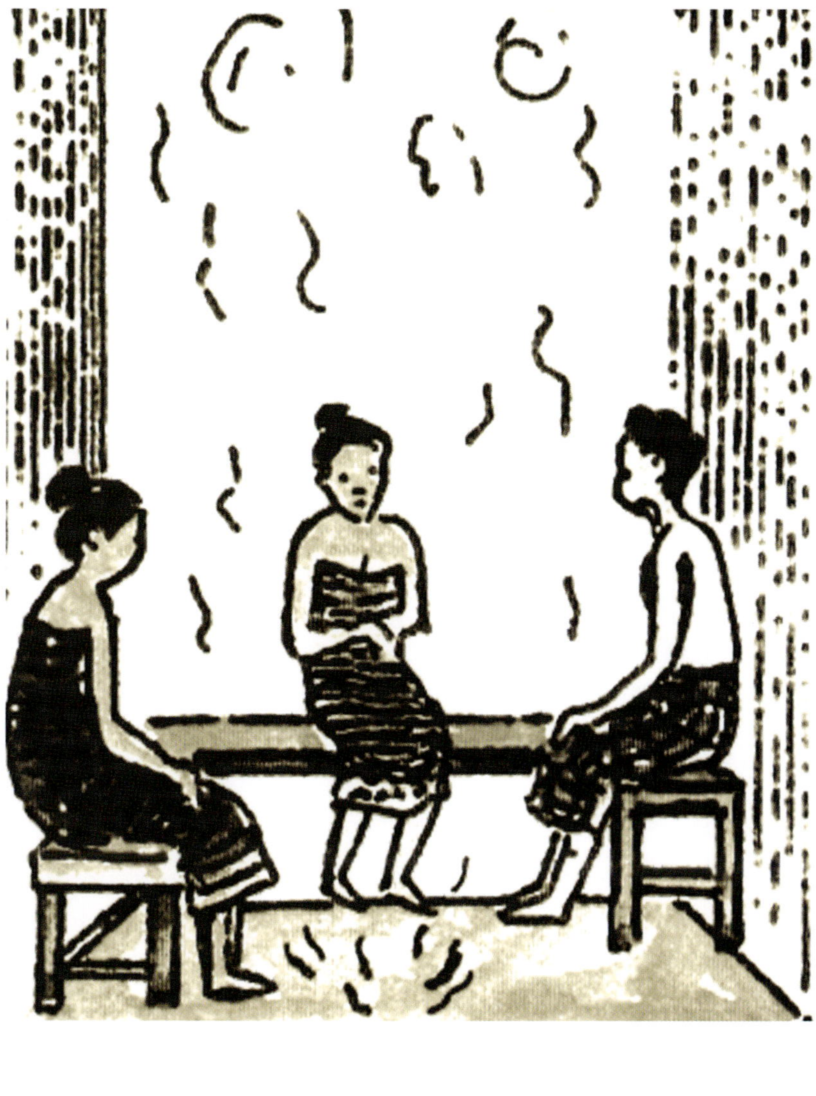

LAO TRADITIONAL MEDICINE

Traditional healing methods in Laos are a perfect example of this blend of early Indian medical practice and regional folk traditions. Lao traditional doctors have developed a holistic system that seeks to restore harmony, either within the individual, between the individual and his or her community, or with their environment. Contemporary healers often specialize in particular areas of medicine such as herbal preparations, massage, bone setting, psychological counselling or even exorcism and magic. Others perform shamanic rituals on behalf of the community, to restore balance, or to bring rain and a bountiful harvest. Local practitioners are still very popular because their cures are often cheaper and more accessible than western allopathic medicine. They also show sensitivity to their native culture and beliefs, incorporating community wisdom into their assessment of each patient and their health situation.

According to the Indian model, physical illnesses is attributed to imbalances in the four elements of nature; earth, air, fire and water, which are reflected in the human body.

1. The earth element controls all the structural or solid aspects of the body, including the internal organs and skeleton.
2. The wind element relates to breathing, bodily movement and to all the air circulating throughout the body systems.
3. The Fire Element relates to the life force, or vital energy, and heat in the body. It also represents the "fire" that causes emotional distress and premature aging.
4. Lastly, the water element relates to all liquids, phlegm and semi solid aspects of the body, such as blood and fat.

During consultations traditional physicians analyze the relative strengths and weaknesses within these elements in a patient's body, calculating how to restore balance. Imbalances in the elements can be aggravated by age, psychological or social factors, diet and exercise, or by emotional and environmental stresses. Because of their holistic view towards the causes of disease, prescribing appropriate medications is often combined with counselling or advice on lifestyle changes, to stimulate the patient's own participation in the healing process.

Medications are formulated from a large selection of natural pharmaceuticals and some herbalists are exceptionally knowledgeable in their field. During their apprenticeship, students learn where medicines come from and how they should look, taste and smell. They also study when and how ingredients should be harvested.

Ingredients are divided into two categories, those that taste cold, hot or gentle, and those that are bitter, fragrant, sweet, astringent, nauseating, nutty, pungent, salty or sour.

Personalized prescriptions are drawn up by combining four types of ingredients:

1. The main drug with the core active ingredient to treat the disease.
2. Other drugs, which might boost the effect of the main drug or help to maintain a balance between the four elements during the healing process.
3. Additives to control the toxicity of the drugs or to enhance or even limit their effectiveness.
4. Additional flavourings and colourings to make the medication more attractive or more palatable.

Treatments involve the participation of friends and family at all stages of the healing process.

To be successful, it is said that herbalists must develop purity of mind, body and action, and be respectful towards their own teachers. It is not uncommon to find Buddhist monks and nuns who are practicing herbalists or for Buddhist monasteries to offer health services to both the monastic and lay communities. This is particularly true of the monks and nuns of the Lao Forest Tradition of Theravada Buddhism, who are well known for their skill in meditation and their deep knowledge of herbal cures. It is said that some of them can even make a diagnosis, and discover a suitable method of treatment, through insights gained during meditation. Forest monasteries frequently have a resident monk doctor who is responsible for the preparation of pills and other traditional medications. He might also include psychological counselling or the use of sacred Buddhist chants to heal the sick.

Nuns are also active herbalists and many specialize in the use of aromatic plants for the prevention and cure of disease. This area of medicine is known today as Aromatherapy and has, since the time of the Buddha, been encouraged as a method for promoting health in the community. According to ancient Buddhist texts, there are four main kinds of Aromatherapy treatments that can be offered in a monastery; these are: herbal steam baths, herbal water baths, teas or infusions, and finally pills. Secondary treatments might include: herbal compresses, ointments and balms, or massage (administered by lay massage therapists).

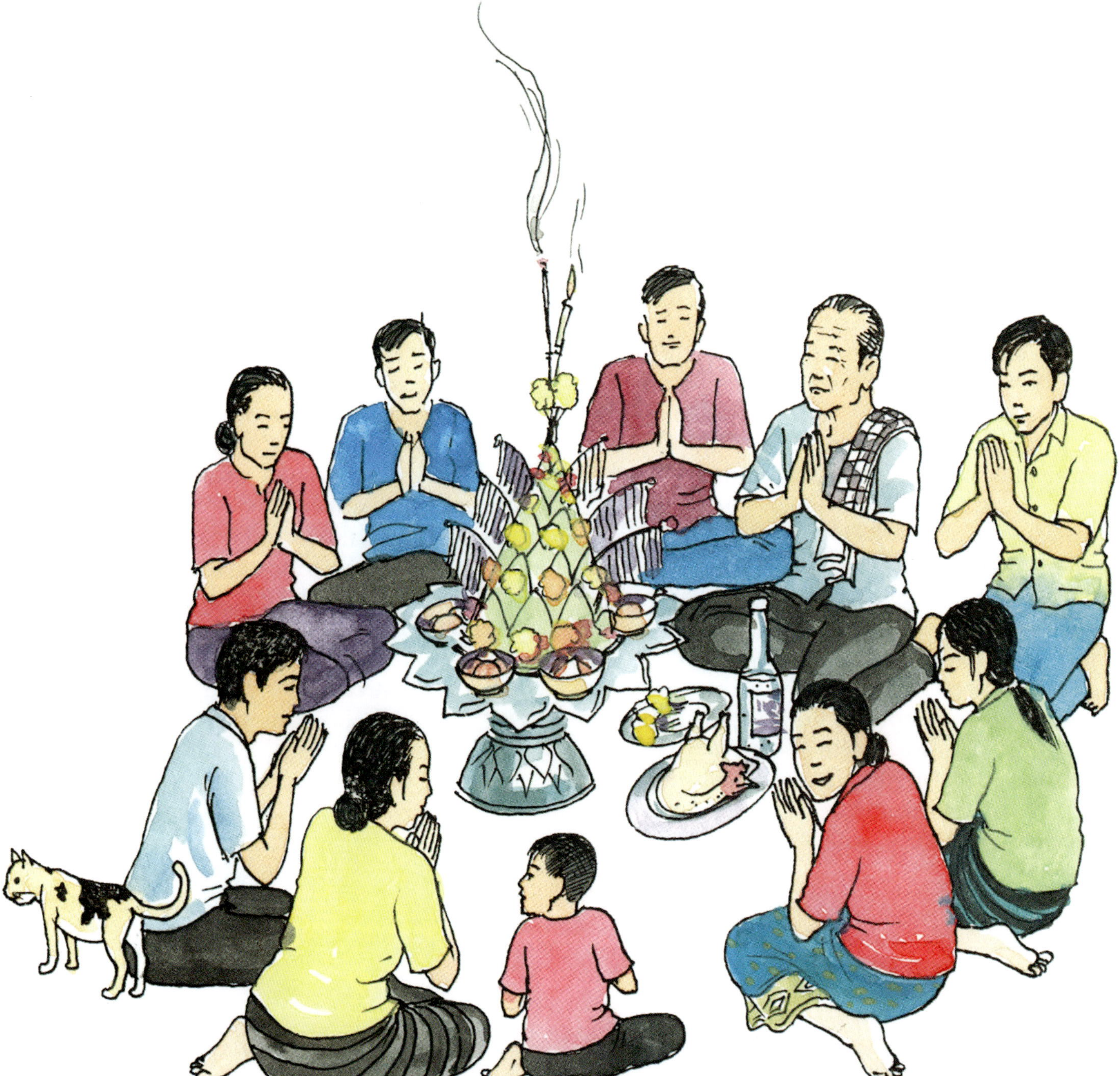

BACI

The Baci is a ritual from the Lao folk tradition. It is generally performed for an individual or a group who are undergoing changes in their lives or to celebrate a special event. A lay practitioner, who knows the ritual chants and who has prepared himself with fasting and purification, leads the ceremony.

Lao people believe a person's body houses 32 vital energies, one relating to each bodily faculty or organ. It is widely held that at times of major change, travel or in times of physical or emotional ill health, one's consciousness becomes unstable and some of the vital energies stray away from the body altogether. These "energies", they say, have a tendency to wander and this is perhaps the feeling we have when we say we feel "scattered", "un-together", "all over the place" or "off-center". At such times the family and friends of the affected person, or group, gather together to offer their support by performing a Baci. The ceremony is designed to rebalance the vital energies and everyone attending is connected by white cotton threads originating from a central alter. This ceremony can also be used as a preventative measure, to minimize the escape of the vital energies and to symbolize the connection between the participants and the spirit world. Traditional offerings, such as money, candles, food and flowers are placed on the alter, then prayers are said and chants are sung to create harmony and balance for those present. At the end everyone ties white cotton stings on the wrists of everyone else while verbalizing their best wishes and the blessings of prosperity and good fortune on all the participants. A feast of chicken, eggs, sweets and local alcohol follows to celebrate the success of the ceremony.

Buddhist monks may be invited to bless such a gathering but will not remain to participate in the ceremony itself, which they feel is rooted in spiritualism more than in Buddhist beliefs. Also the serving of alcohol is against their monastic vows.

CLINICAL AROMATHERAPY

Most people have already heard of Aromatherapy as it is used in beauty treatments and perfumery, but are less familiar with its origins, which are deeply rooted in traditional medicine. When applied to healing, it is more accurately known as Clinical Aromatherapy. Aromatic plants can prevent disease, treat illness and enhance harmony in the body and mind. They do this through their active constituents known as essential oils. These oils are called "essential" because they represent the essence of the plant from which they are obtained. In modern times essential oils have been chemically tested and found to be a complex mixture of organic compounds; primarily terpenes, esters, aldehydes, ketones, alcohols, phenols and oxides. There are about 30,000 known compounds in essential oils, which are found in oil-bearing leaves, flowers, bark, seeds, or the wood of aromatic plants. They are used in healing, beauty products, perfumery and food flavourings. A few of the important constituents in essential oils have been chemically synthesized but they lack the subtle odours and curative properties present in the natural oils. The complex mixtures of trace elements, sometimes several hundred in a single oil, have so far proved impossible to duplicate. Essential oils can be released from aromatic plants and extracted by various methods. Steam distillation, however, is the most common method of extraction and is the method used, for example, in herbal steam baths.

Essential oils have valuable medicinal properties that have both physiological and psychological effects. Physiologically they act directly on the organs and body systems, while psychologically they act on the mind through the sense of smell. The sense of smell is linked to the limbic system of the brain, which is the seat of emotion and memory. It is through this connection that fragrances affect our mood and stimulate memories. Once ingested, essential oils pass through the body and are eliminated through the lungs, urine and the skin.

The Body

Human beings are among the most complex organisms in the world. Billions of microscopic parts, each with its own identity, work together in an organized manner for the benefit of the whole being. The human body is a single structure but it is made up of billions of smaller structures of four major kinds: cells, which are the simplest units of living matter and can reproduce themselves; tissues, which are organizations of many similar cells with nonliving, intercellular substances between them; organs, organizations of several different kinds of tissues arranged together to perform a specific function; and body systems, which are the most complex component units in the human body. They comprise an organization of different numbers and kinds of organs that are arranged in such a way that they can perform complex functions for the body. There are ten major body systems; cardiovascular, skeletal, muscular, lymphatic, respiratory, digestive, reproductive, urinary, endocrine and nervous. There are also other important systems, like the immune system, and many organs, such as the skin, which are beneficially affected by the use of essential oils.

The cardio-vascular system or *circulatory system* consists of the heart, the vessels that transport blood to and from the heart, and the spleen. The spleen breaks down worn out red blood corpuscles and also acts as a reservoir for blood. A healthy spleen contracts every twenty or thirty seconds and this has some influence on the blood pressure. Plant oils affect the circulatory systems directly by lowering or stimulating blood pressure.

Although *the skeletal system* is not directly affected by the presence of essential oils in the bloodstream the related *muscular system* benefits greatly from the oils, particularly those that have a warming or cooling effect. They improve blood circulation and provide pain relief to the muscles and joints through their analgesic or anti-inflammatory effects. Treatment can be given via teas and tinctures, inhalation, compresses over the heart area and with aromatic baths.

The lymphatic system consists of tissues and organs, including bone marrow, spleen, thymus, and lymph nodes, that produce and store lymphocytes or cells that fight infection, as well as the channels that carry lymph fluid. The entire lymphatic system is an important part of the body's immune system. It disposes of unwanted waste from the body and battles infections. Treatment of the lymphatic system can be given orally, by using compresses over the heart and by taking aromatic baths.

The respiratory system is made up of the organs that process air in the body, including the nose, throat and lungs. Respiratory problems of all kinds respond very well to treatment with essential oils, particularly though steam inhalation, as they cause an increase in bronchial secretions and are readily absorbed into the blood stream. This is due to their antispasmodic, antiseptic and expectorant actions. Their ability to treat colds and flu is well known but they are also effective against other respiratory infections such as whooping cough and in the treatment of asthma. When treating respiratory complaints essential oils are taken by inhalation, by local compresses or orally.

The digestive system is comprised of the organs that take in food and turn it into energy that the body can use to stay healthy. Waste products that the body cannot use leave the body through bowel movements. The digestive system includes the salivary glands, mouth, esophagus, stomach, liver, pancreas, gallbladder, small and large intestines, and rectum. The aroma of tasty food stimulates the digestive juices. Once we taste the food the production of saliva is stimulated and this further stimulates the digestive juices. Although we think of tasting as taking place in the mouth, much of what we think of as flavour is experienced via the sense of smell. The mouth is only able to register four basic tastes, salty, sour, sweet and bitter. The more tasty the food and more importantly, the better it smells, the better we digest it. Many of the aromatic spices and herbs, which we add to food to enhance its flavour, also aid digestion, calm the stomach and prevent spasms. This is because of the essential oils they contain. Although the digestive system can benefit by essential oils taken in via the skin or by inhalation, treatment is more effective when taken orally such as in the form of medicinal teas, herbal tinctures or in the form of pills. It is also common to use compresses directly onto the stomach area or abdomen.

The reproductive system is responsible for the generation of offspring and includes the ovaries, uterus, vagina, testes and penis. The reproductive organs are affected by the absorption of oils in the bloodstream. Some oils strengthen the system as a whole, while others treat specific ailments such as menstrual irregularity, infections and sexual difficulties. They are also widely used to assist in childbirth. Oils are best introduced into the body through compresses to the abdomen and lower back, herbal hipbaths or orally.

The urinary system produces and releases urine. It includes the kidneys, bladder, and urethra. Problems in the urinary system are not much affected by the inhalation of essential oils. They are best treated orally in teas and tinctures to combat ailments in these areas. It is also possible to use local compresses and hipbaths filled with suitable herbal waters.

The endocrine system is comprised of ductless glands that regulate bodily functions via hormones secreted into the bloodstream. It includes the hypothalamus, pituitary gland, thyroid, adrenal glands, and gonads (ovaries and testes). Essential oils are known to influence the secretion of hormones in the body and therefore can have a profound effect on the health. Firstly they stimulate the endocrine glands, normalizing hormonal secretions. Secondly they act as quasi-hormones themselves. The thyroid gland, which deals with growth and metabolism, the adrenal medulla which deals with stress reactions and the adrenal cortex which governs the production of sex hormones are all benefited by essential oils. Since endocrine disturbance is manifested in almost every type of disease, the possibility of treating it with essential oils is of great interest. In the case of endocrine malfunction the oils are best ingested either by inhalation, bathing or in teas.

The nervous system consists of the cells, tissues and organs that regulate the body's responses to internal and external stimuli. It is made up of the brain, spinal cord, nerves, ganglia and neurotransmitters. Many essential oils are known to have either a sedative effect or a stimulating effect on the central nervous system, while others have a balancing effect. This affects the emotions and the general wellbeing of the physical body as well, since they are highly interconnected. Both stress and lethargy are known to have an adverse effect on the body. Aromatherapy can also be used to treat some types of mental illness and have fewer side effects than many allopathic drugs; however, they should be used in conjunction with counselling, psychotherapy and spiritual guidance.

Another system which benefits greatly from Aromatherapy is *the immune system*, which is responsible for fighting disease. Its primary function is to identify foreign substances in the body (bacteria, viruses, fungi or parasites) and develop a defense against them. This defense is known as the immune response. It involves the production of protein molecules called antibodies that eliminate the foreign organisms that invade the body. Almost all essential oils have bactericidal properties and many also promote the production of white blood cells, which can help to prevent and treat infectious diseases. These oils are nature's immune system boosters and their value in this area cannot be over emphasized.

The skin is the natural protective covering of the body and its largest organ. It plays an important role in the absorption of medicinal plant oils during herbal bathing or when essential oils are used in massage, as well as in balms, ointments and compresses. The skin itself is a barometer of the general health of a patient. Skin problems can be seen as manifestations of deeper health problems such as a build up of toxins in the blood, stress or hormonal imbalances. Due to their anti-inflammatory, bactericidal and fungicidal properties, essential oils can heal many skin conditions.

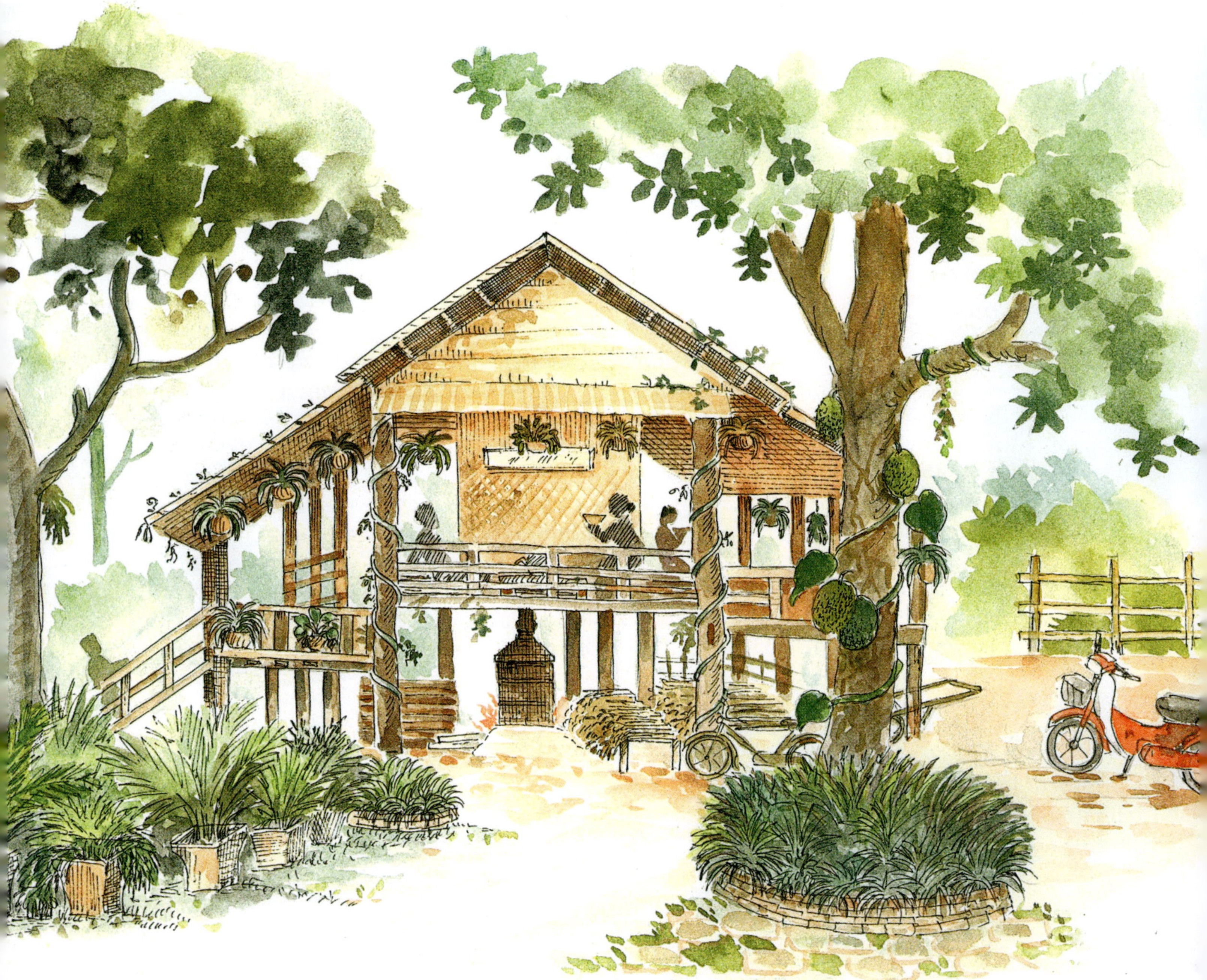

HERBAL AND AROMATHERAPY TREATMENTS

The herbal steam bath

Herbal steam baths are used all over Laos for healing, relaxation and detoxification. In the Lao language herbal steaming is known as *hom yaa* or "fragrant medicine", on account of the aromatic herbs used in its preparations. The benefits of aromatic steaming are well known to Lao people, who frequently drop in for a steam on the way home from work or on the weekends. People who take steam treatments regularly find that they rarely become ill, maintaining good health and spirits. The monastic community also uses the steam room, particularly in the evenings after the lay people have gone home, to promote robust health and treat common ailments.

Steam therapy involves placing fresh and dried aromatic plant parts into boiling water and relaxing in the resulting steam. The steam is heavy with volatile essential oil molecules that are released from the aromatic plants and herbs. These healing chemicals are readily absorbed into the body systems, mainly via inhalation. Steam bath recipes contain carefully blended plants and have been passed down through generations of healers. The blending and quantities of ingredients necessitates an intimate knowledge of both herbal and aromatic medicine. In addition to this the healer needs to be familiar with local plants and their uses, as well as the methods and times of successful harvesting.

During a visit to the *hom yaa*, essential oils can be assimilated by the body in several ways; via the respiratory tract during steam bath inhalation, through the skin in herbal bathing and orally in the form of teas and tinctures. The most effective combination is steam bathing and sipping herbal teas. While enjoying the heat and relaxation of the steam room, it is important to inhale and exhale steadily to maximize the absorption of the essential oils. The airborne molecules in the steam are readily absorbed by the mucus membranes of the respiratory tract and through the surface capillaries in the nose and mouth. In this way they quickly enter the blood stream and body systems. Surprisingly, essential oils are not readily absorbed into the body through the skin during steam bathing, as the body will be sweating and throwing off toxins, rather than absorbing. Absorption through the skin can take place only when the body is not sweating; therefore some people like to leave trace oils on the skin after steaming and do not shower for several hours after the body has cooled, allowing time for absorbtion.

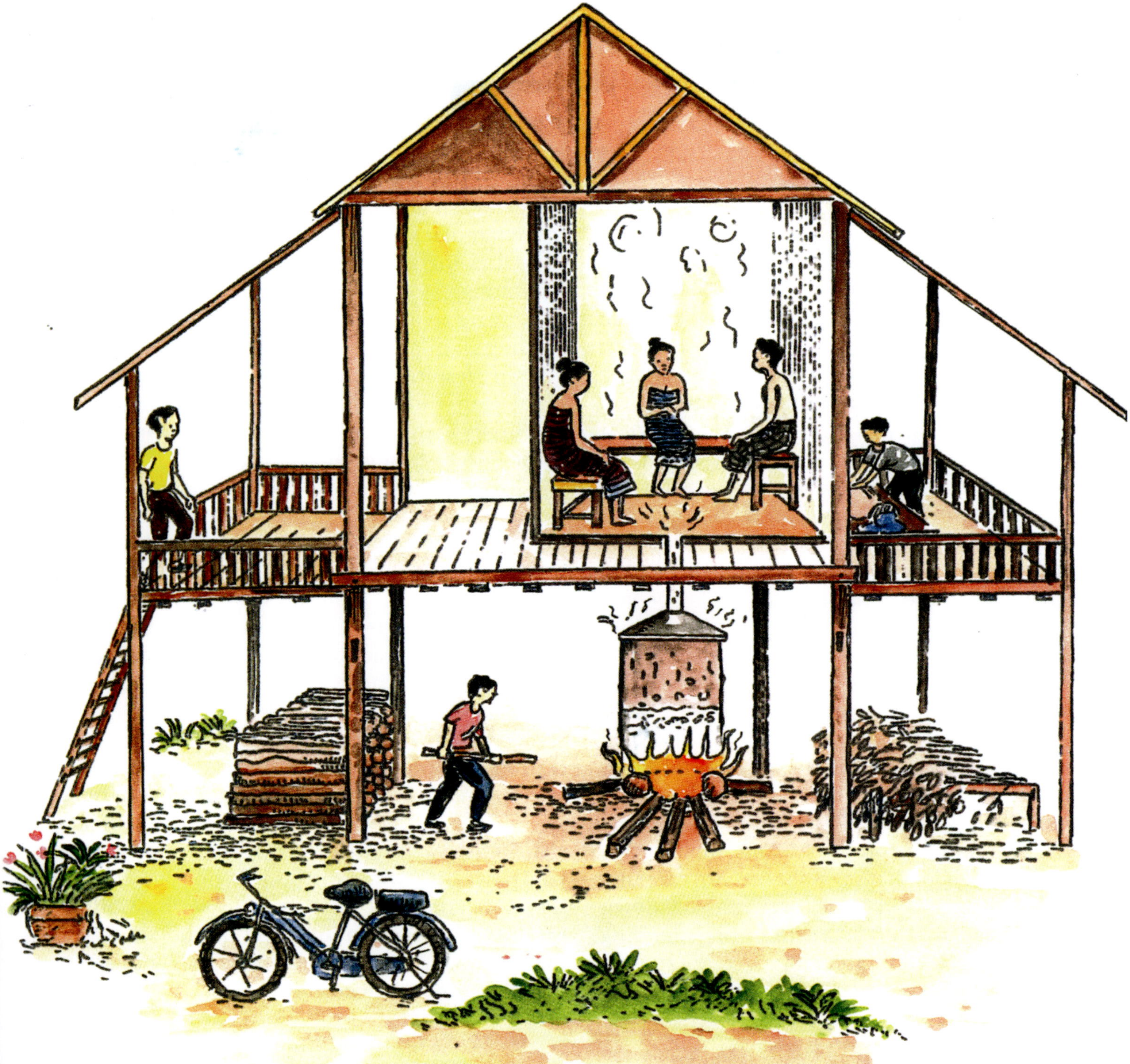

Construction of a herbal steam room

The traditional architecture of Laos lends itself perfectly to the creation of herbal steam baths, as the rural houses are built on stilts. Such houses are constructed primarily of indigenous hardwoods, which grow in the tropical forests and the open space below the building allows for a multitude of uses. In the case of aromatic steam house buildings, it allows a dry space for the storage of medicinal plants and a suitable area to build an apparatus for creating steam.

The apparatus used to create the steam is thus placed below the building and consists of a water drum that is placed on top of a fireplace made of rocks and mud. This allows for a fire to be built under the drum. There is a small opening near the top of the drum through which fresh water and medicinal plants can be introduced, and a drainage hole in the bottom to drain off used herbal waters and plant matter. Lastly, a large sealed pipe runs from the top of the drum up through a hole in the wooden floor of the house above, allowing steam to rise directly from the drum and into the steam room.

Each day, fresh water is poured into the drum and a fire is lit beneath it. Once the water is boiling, a bundle of carefully selected medicinal plants is dropped directly into the water through the small opening in the top of the drum. As the plants heat up and boil, their volatile essential oils are released and carried upwards through the pipe in the form of aromatic steam to the room above. The steam room itself is enclosed except for the pipe hole in its floor and a door. A curtain is usually drawn across the inside of the door to minimize the escape of steam as people move in and out. Narrow wooden benches are placed along the walls of the room for clients to sit on while they sweat and inhale the medicinal vapors that rise up from below. This simple system creates a most effective steam room.

Herbal ingredients

Herbal steam bath formulas differ somewhat from region to region based on the availability of plants and the personal preferences of the practitioner. Due to their familiarity with local plants, healers can adapt ancient recipes to suit regional conditions. In addition many healers cultivate plants in their own botanical gardens, particularly those that are used in large quantities, for ease and convenience. In spite of this, it is not possible to cultivate all the necessary plants and some must still be collected from the forests and fields. Great care goes into selection of the ingredients and the recipes are frequently kept secret. The collection of wild herbal ingredients requires great expertise and is a dying art. Certain locations, which produce superior plants, are carefully identified due perhaps to the soil quality or climatic conditions. Harvesting must also be timed precisely. For example the moon is said to have an effect on the medicinal potency of plants and the quality of their essential oils, so certain phases of the moon are selected for harvesting. Similarly, the time of day can play an important role. While harvesting, traditional plant collectors are required to perform ritual chants and make offerings to the spirits of nature. They request permission to pick the plants, asking for protection and blessings for themselves and for the patients who will use them. It is believed that these practices enhance the healing power of the plants on a subtle or energetic level and help prevent negative influences from contaminating the medicines.

Many herbalists in Laos are still fortunate enough to have access to fresh ingredients for their recipes. In the more urbanized parts of the region however, it has become necessary to use dried plants, or to substitute plants that are no longer available in the diminishing forests. Fresh, as opposed to dried, plants are preferred, because many of the therapeutic volatile oils and trace elements are lost in the drying process. The loss of chemical constituents can adversely affect the efficacy of the blend. Therefore, to provide full therapeutic value, it is of great benefit to have fresh and well-harvested plants.

Preparation of the herbal ingredients

Once the plants have been appropriately gathered they are sorted, cleaned and selected for blending. Sauna plants seem to be selected on the basis of their individual medicinal properties, rather than on possible synergistic effects they may exhibit when combined with other plants, although there are some exceptions to this rule.

Quantities for a daily sauna blend are simply a handful of each plant and half as much of the stronger or more pungent plants, like Camphor, Basil or Eucalyptus. Once measured, the plants are tied in a cotton bundle and placed into the boiling water to provide medicinal vapors to the room above.

For daily use in the steam room, plants that prevent disease and promote relaxation are generally chosen, since they are beneficial for most people. The plants used on a regular basis do differ a little from day to day, and season to season, depending on the availability of quality plants.

In the case of acute conditions, or more serious illnesses, special prescriptions are prepared for a personal steam bath. In such cases, if the problem is caught early enough, it is not uncommon for the patient to make a full recovery without the need for stronger medications. Herbal steam bathing is also effective for many chronic ailments, as well as after childbirth and in convalescence. Since the main purpose of herbal steam bathing is to introduce essential oils into the systems of the body and to detect the fragrances of the plants, it is best to be in the steam room when the plants have recently been introduced. In this case however, the eyes should be kept closed, as this is when the steam is most saturated with oil molecules and they can irritate the delicate tissues of the eyes. Most good steam bath managers change the plants several times per day.

INHALATION

In addition to its physical benefits, the steam room offers subtle healing to the emotions and to the mind. It offers this through the aromas of the healing plants. Scientific investigation has shown that fragrance has a direct effect on certain areas of the brain through the sense of smell, or process of olfaction. This process is very complex and allows us to differentiate aromas with only slightly different chemical constituents. Human beings can distinguish over 10,000 aromas, which effect our mood, bring back memories and can calm or stimulate our minds. Appealing aromas are very personal and everyone has their own personal likes and dislikes whether in food, perfume or incense.

The olfactory bulb is part of the limbic system of the brain and is related to our ability to learn and remember, as well as to our emotions and sexuality. The aromatic molecules in plants stimulate receptor cells in the nasal cavity that send electrical impulses to the olfactory bulb in the brain and this in turn activates enzyme production. The limbic system is also the link between the voluntary and involuntary nervous systems, as well as the left and right brain. Exactly how these chemicals enter and work on the brain is still the subject of scientific study but this much we know, the aromas inhaled during the steam baths effect the mind as well as treat the body.

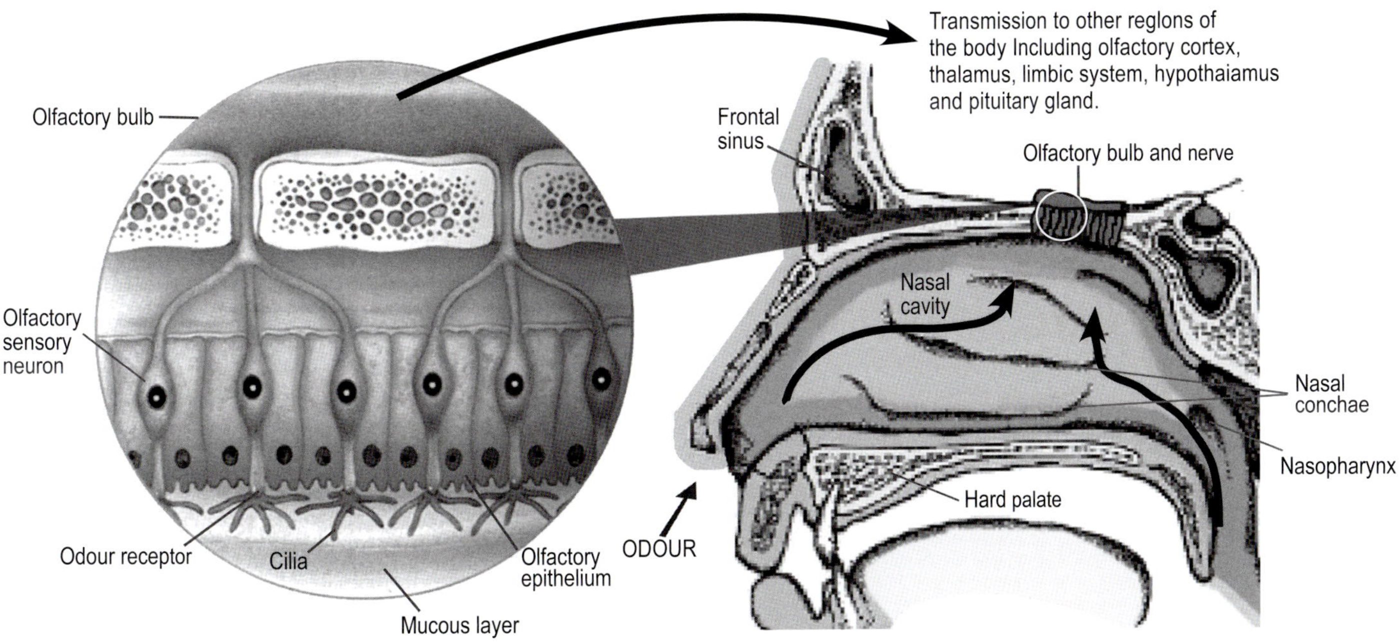

Herbal Water Bath

At the end of each day herbal waters remaining in the drum can be drained, strained, cooled and used for bathing. In this case the main organ of absorption is the skin and subtly through the airborne fragrances. When not sweating, the skin provides a highly absorptive surface for plant chemicals to enter the body. In many trials it has been seen that essential oils, or their components, have shown up in the blood, lymph or urine very shortly after being applied to the skin. Clearly essential oils pass through the skin very quickly.

Sometimes the herbal waters are used as a treatment in their own right. This method of bathing in herbal waters predates the use of steam bathing in Laos. The waters are ladled over the body repeatedly and left to dry naturally, leaving those essential oils directly on the skin. Alternatively, one can submerge the whole body in a bath of herbal waters or take a hip bath for certain ailments. Many kinds of herbal bathing have been used for centuries all over the world for therapeutic purposes as well as for pleasure.

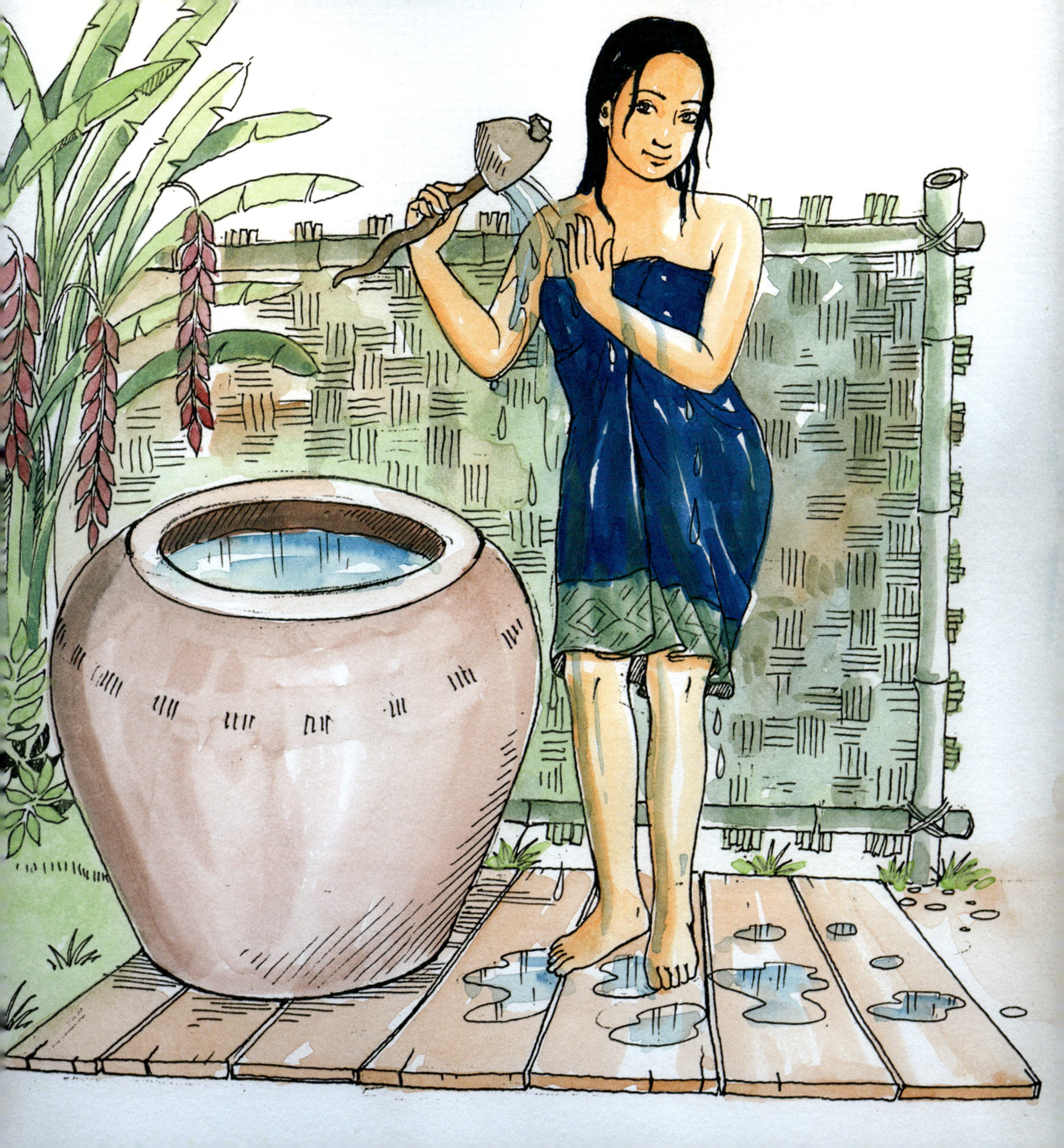

Infusions (teas) and fluid extracts

To supplement the healing effects of the steam room, it is common practice to offer herbal teas to drink while cooling off. The teas include ingredients for general health, to simulate the immune system and to purify the body. Health giving teas are brewed by blending healing plants, pouring hot water over them and leaving the mixture to steep before serving it to the clients. However, in the case of specific ailments, stronger medicinal extracts can be prepared to treat an individual directly. To make a stronger extract, the herbal blend is added to water and boiled for up to half an hour before serving.

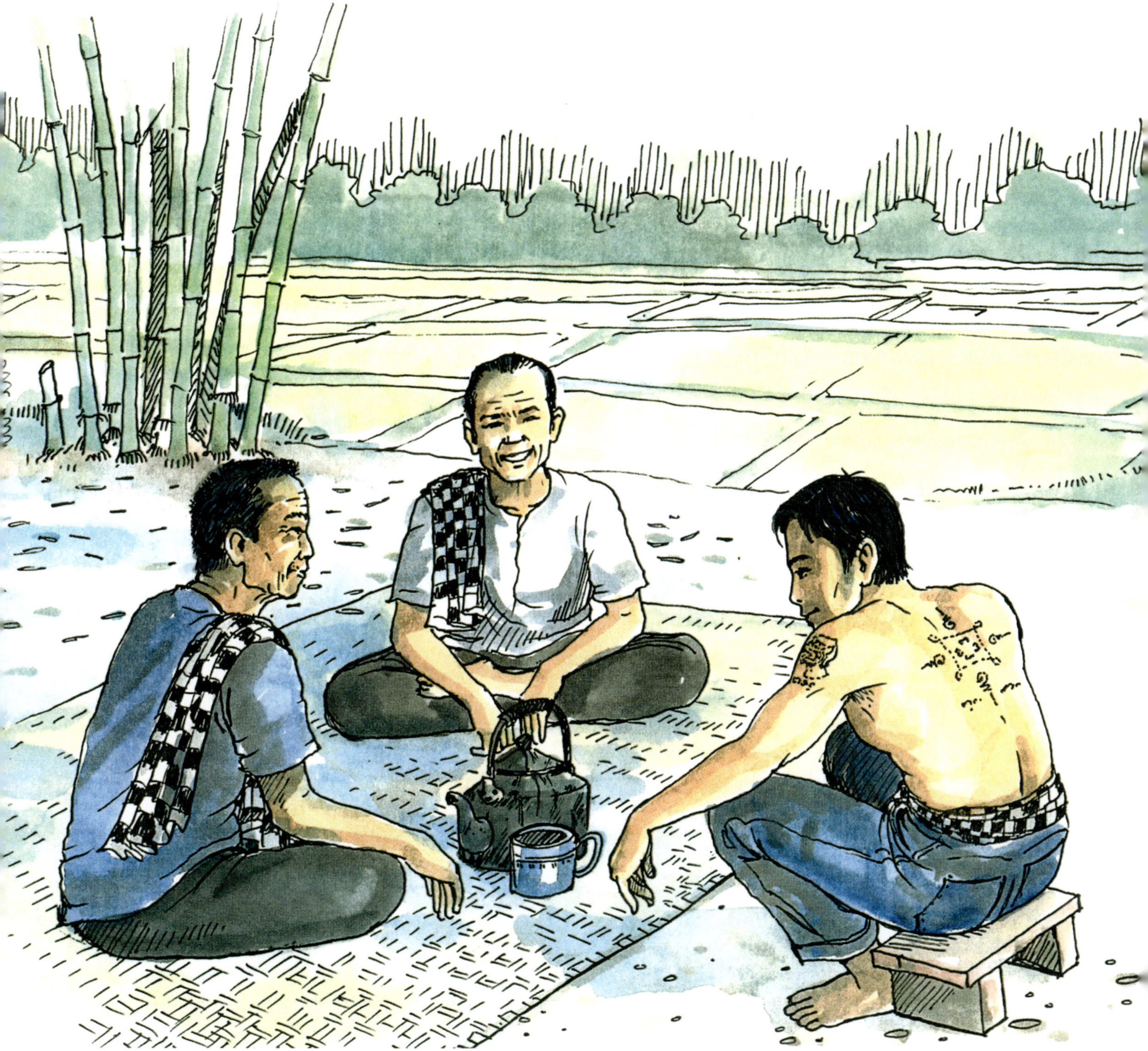

Massage, the power of touch

There are some 50,000,000 touch receptors in the skin and the healing power of touch is known to all over the world. We use the power of touch when we spontaneously hug a friend who is sad, cradle a crying baby in our arms, place our hand on an aching head or reach out to touch someone in need. It is this caring motivation, as we touch another person, which is the single most important aspect of all types of massage therapy. In many families, children are touched openly and affectionately while they are young but this often stops when they reach puberty. As a result teenagers and young adults, who are not married or in a loving relationship, are seldom touched. This is also true of older people or those who are no longer sexually active. The result in all cases is the same—they feel lonely, isolated and unloved—untouched.

A lot of confusion has arisen between "loving touch" and sexual intimacy. To help overcome these social difficulties, many cultures around the world have developed a formalized system of touching called massage. This allows for prolonged and soothing physical contact with another person without the fear of sexual misunderstandings. Loving touch seems fundamental to our sense of wellbeing, especially in the fast moving, modern world in which we live today. What is a little harder to understand is how this contact affects our health and even speeds recovery from serious illnesses, but it does. We all seem drawn to the touch of kind hands. The rising popularity of day spas, beauty parlors and longer-term health treatment centers, that offer various kinds of massage and physical therapy, is based on our need to relax and to be touched. This should hardly be surprising given the habits of our closest relative, the apes, who spend hours each day grooming, touching and hugging each other.

Healing touch can be used to release tensions in the body or mind that can so easily lead to disease. "Dis-ease" describes the state that precedes illness, a lack of ease or harmony in the body or mind. If we can learn to notice this feeling and address it with the healing touch of massage, or other preventative treatments, problems can often be averted. In Laos, massage is commonly shared within families as a kind of social bonding and has been practiced in rural communities for centuries. It is also offered in many village monasteries, by the lay community, as part of their healing services.

Lao style massage follows the Indian system of yoga with its detailed description of invisible energy pathways that form a network throughout the body. It is along such pathways that vital energy, or life force, flows and keeps us alive and well. When these energies are flowing correctly around the pathways, the person experiences good health with a bright and positive mind. If the pathways become obstructed, then the life force becomes imbalanced, causing the body and mind to become disturbed. Such imbalances can lead, not only to physical illness, but to dullness, emotional negativity or even to a severe health crisis.

The technique of Lao massage works on the main energy pathways to remove existing blockages and to help the body reestablish optimal energy flows. This is achieved by applying several techniques; stretching and compressing the muscles, using thumb pressures along the energy pathways or by moving and gently rocking muscles, ligaments and nerves to redirect energy flow. The massage therapist uses hands, knees, feet and elbows to unblock and correct the flow of life force, returning the patient to a sense of harmony and balance. This type of massage does not call for the use of oils and is performed with the patient dressed in loose clothing.

In the Lao monastery, massage is regarded as a spiritual activity. It might begin with a prayer, perhaps a wish to help the person who has come seeking help, and might end with a word of thanks. Massage should be given in a focused and meditative frame of mind, as a simple offering of loving kindness combined with a genuine wish to help. A massage given in this frame of mind has a profound affect, as both masseur and patient are intuitively aware of the subtle communication that is being exchanged through the energy in the hands.

Lao massage also includes deep stretches that feel like having another person perform yoga postures on the body for you, rather than performing them yourself. In the Indian medical tradition, the practice of Yoga postures for health is well established. An authentic massage practitioner would be expected to perform their own physical exercises, meditation and spiritual activities as an example to others and to encourage them in healthy living practices.

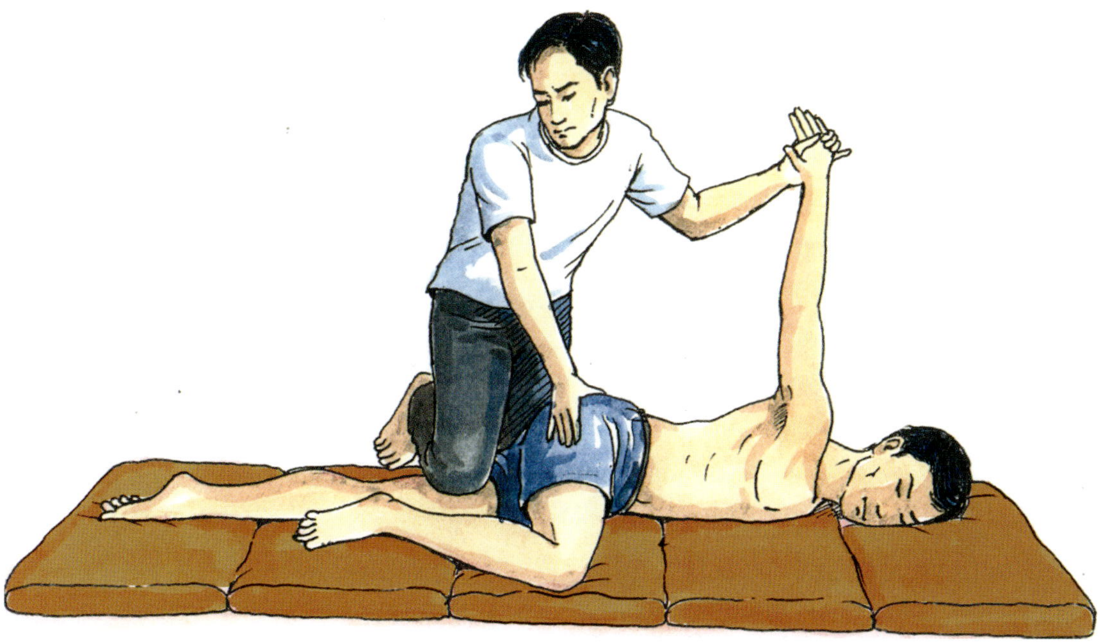

Pills

In the context of monastic medicine, the preparation of pills is often left to monk doctors who are, in general, specialized in the field of diagnosis and the prescription of stronger medications. Of course the making of pills is also practiced by other traditional herbalists as well. To make herbal pills the ingredients are prepared differently to the steam room plants, which are chopped, shredded or crushed. For the preparation of pills the ingredients are dried and ground into a powder. The powder is bound by adding honey until a dough is formed. The dough is then kneaded and shaped into small balls before being sun-dried. Such pills last for up to a month in sealed jars and are best used fresh.

Compresses

Another therapy offered at the Lao sauna is that of herbal compresses. These compresses are prepared by wrapping freshly chopped or ground herbs, and other aromatic ingredients, in a small cotton cloth bag and tying it into a ball. The ball is then steam heated before applying it to the body. The compress is about the size of a grapefruit and, after warming, is applied by rolling it on the affected area. Herbal balls are used to reduce muscular tension, aches and pains, inflammation in the joints or skin, bruising, fatigue and cramps. It also prevents muscular atrophy due to various kinds of paralysis and is nourishing to the skin. The intense heat reduces water retention and encourages dilation of capillaries, which assists in the absorption of the essential oils in the herbs; it also helps increase the blood circulation and relieves congestion in the respiratory system. Compresses are also said to open blocked energy channels, to detoxify the body and to relieve stress or depression through their aromatic effects. Herbs are chosen according to symptoms.

THE FRAGRANT PLANTS

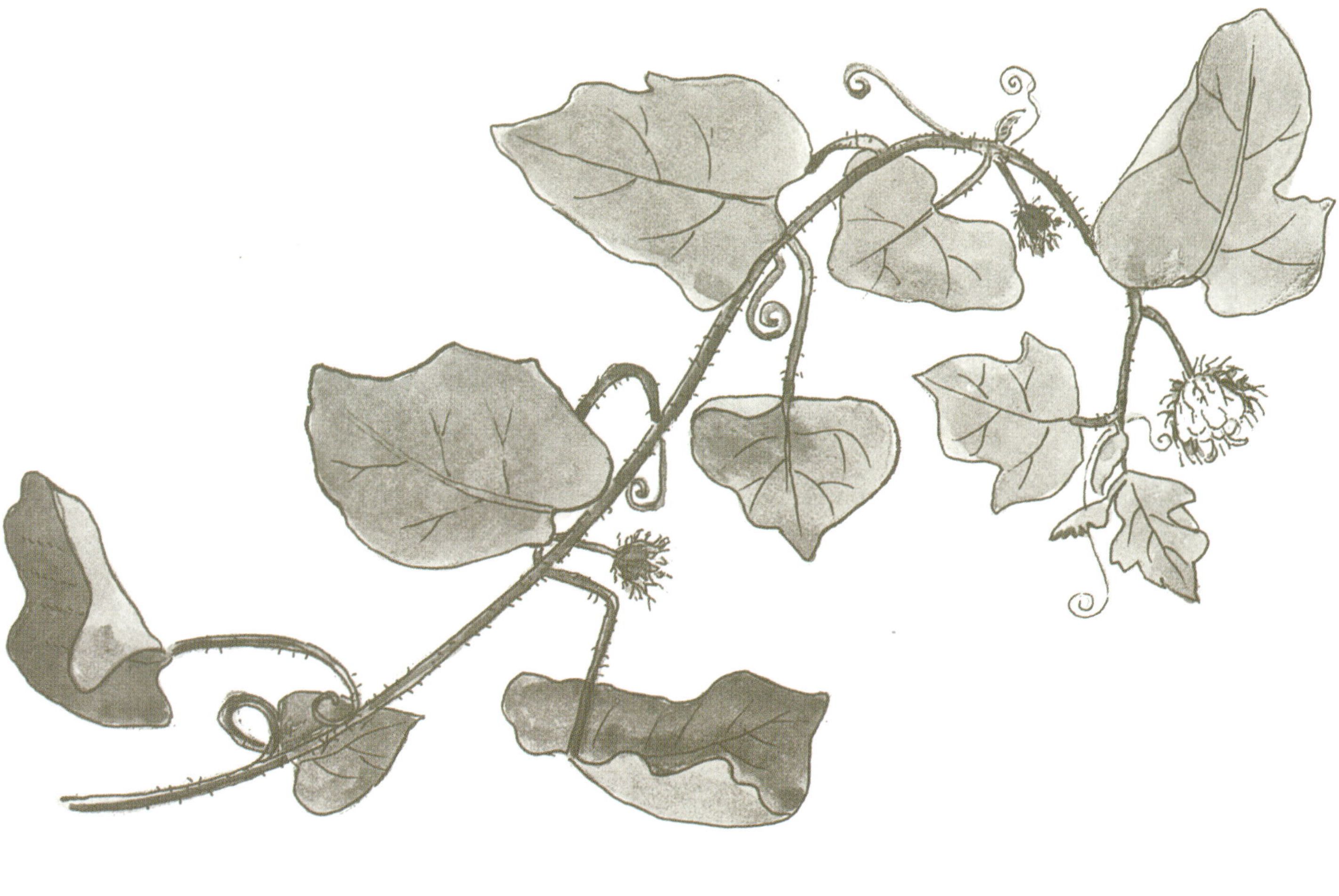

I. PLANTS USED DAILY

1. *Adenosma bracteosum Bon.*

Family: *Scrophulariaceae*

English name: ——

Vernacular name / Local name: *i-tuu naa* or *ji-naai kohrm*

Name in Lao script: ອີ່ຕູ່ນາ, ຈີ່ນາຍກ້ອມ

Part used in saunas: whole plant with flowers

Description:

A perennial herb, 30-50 cm in height, that occurs naturally in rice paddy fields. The stem and branch are tetragonal with few ramifications at node. Leaves are lanceolate, 2-3 cm long, occurring opposite at node. Inflorescence is in a very dense terminal spike. The whole plant is strongly fragrant.

Benefits:

I-ttu naa is used in abundance at the sauna in its matured dried state. Its very strong scent is good for respiratory ailments, herbal bathing after childbirth, analgesic, anti-inflammatory, skin beauty.

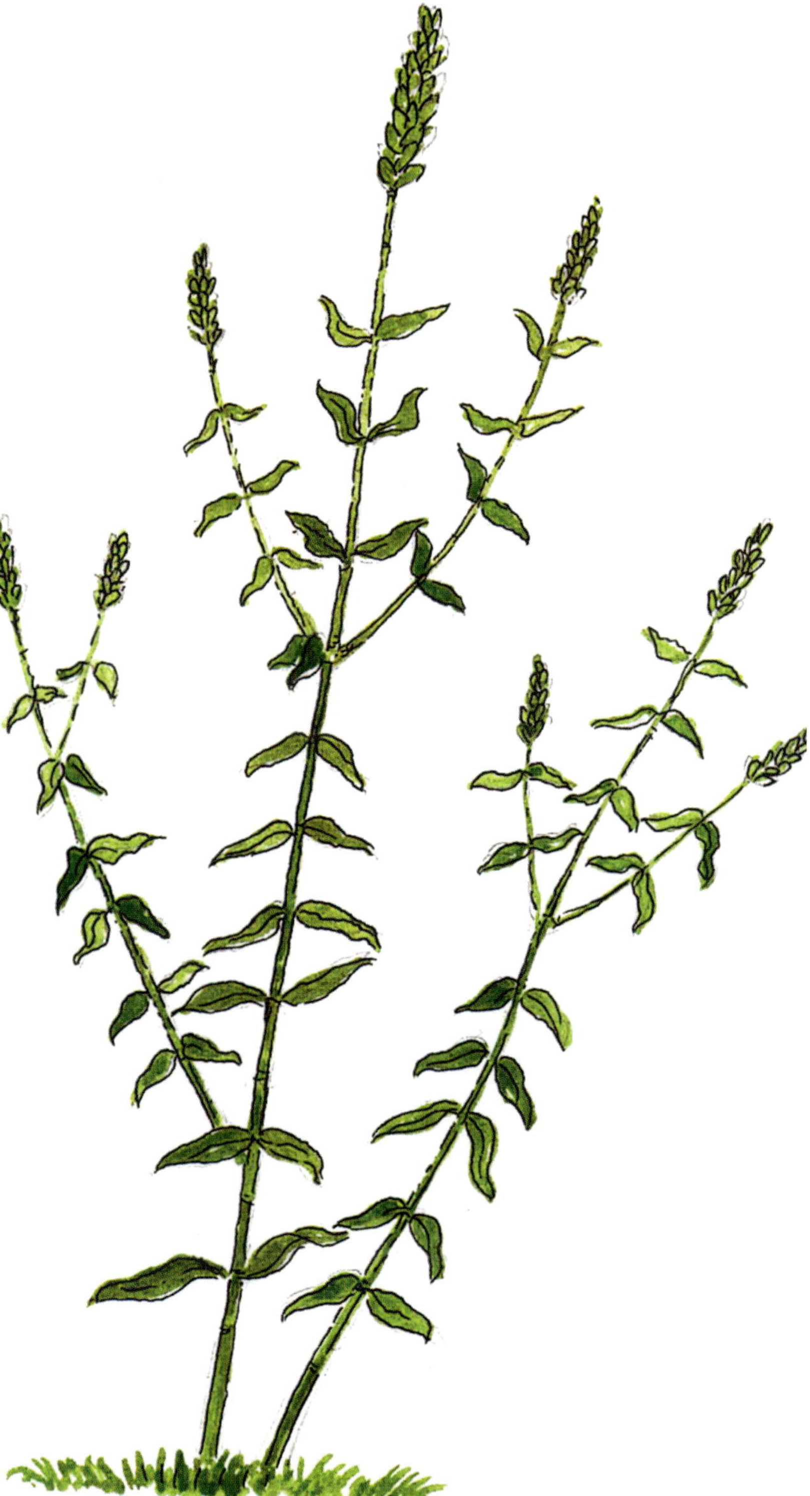

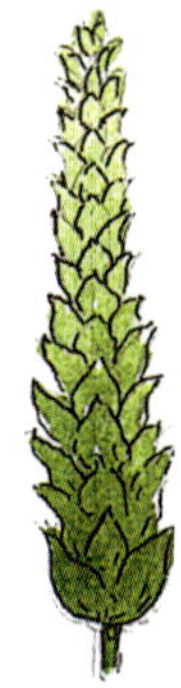

2. *Blumea balsamifera (Linn.)* DC.

Family: *Asteraceae*

English name: Camphor tree

Vernacular name /Local name: *ton naat nyai,ton naat luang*

Name in Lao script: ຕົ້ນໜາດໃຫຍ່, ຕົ້ນໜາດຫຼວງ

Part used in saunas: leaves

Description:

A shrub 2-3 m tall. The stem is soft, green and velutinous when young, becoming brownish with maturity. The leaves are lanceolate and velutinous, 6-8 cm wide and 20-25 cm long, in a spiral arrangement. The petiole is about 5 cm long, bearing two to three pairs of leaves. Excrescence on the two edge lines of the upper surface. The inflorescence is in the axillary and terminal heads, with a panicle of yellow flowers. The whole plant is highly scented.

Benefits:

Heartburn & indigestion, treats insomnia, hypertension, antispasmodic, stimulates sweating, respiratory ailments & asthma, antibacterial, stomach problems, headaches, dizziness, joint pains.

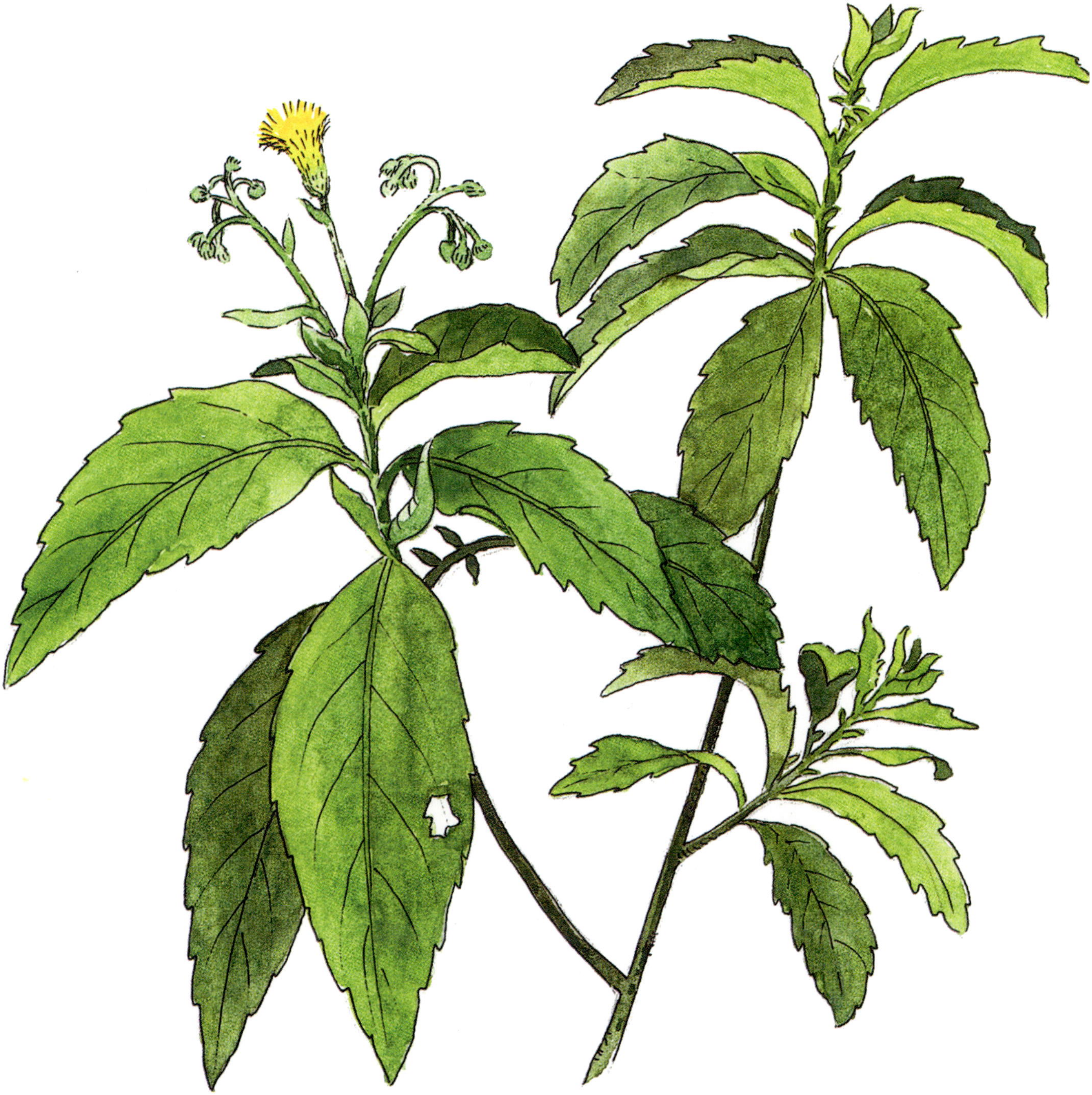

3. *Citrus hystrix DC.*

Family: *Rutaceae*

English name: Leech lime

Vernacular name / Local name: *ton khi-huut*

Name in Lao script: ຕົ້ນຂີ້ຫູດ

Part used in saunas: leaves

Description:

A small tree 2-8 m in height, with strong thorny stems and twigs. The arrangement of leaves is alternate. The leaves are a bright, dark green with a wing almost the same size as the leaf itself. Both are oblong with a rounded apex and have a strong scent. The flowers are white and fragrant with multiple blooms 1 cm in length. The fruit is about 5 cm in height with a thick crinkled skin, which has a strong citrus scent. The flesh of the fruit is sour and slightly bitter.

Benefits:

Stimulant, stomach ache, blood purifier, good for hair & skin, respiratory congestion.

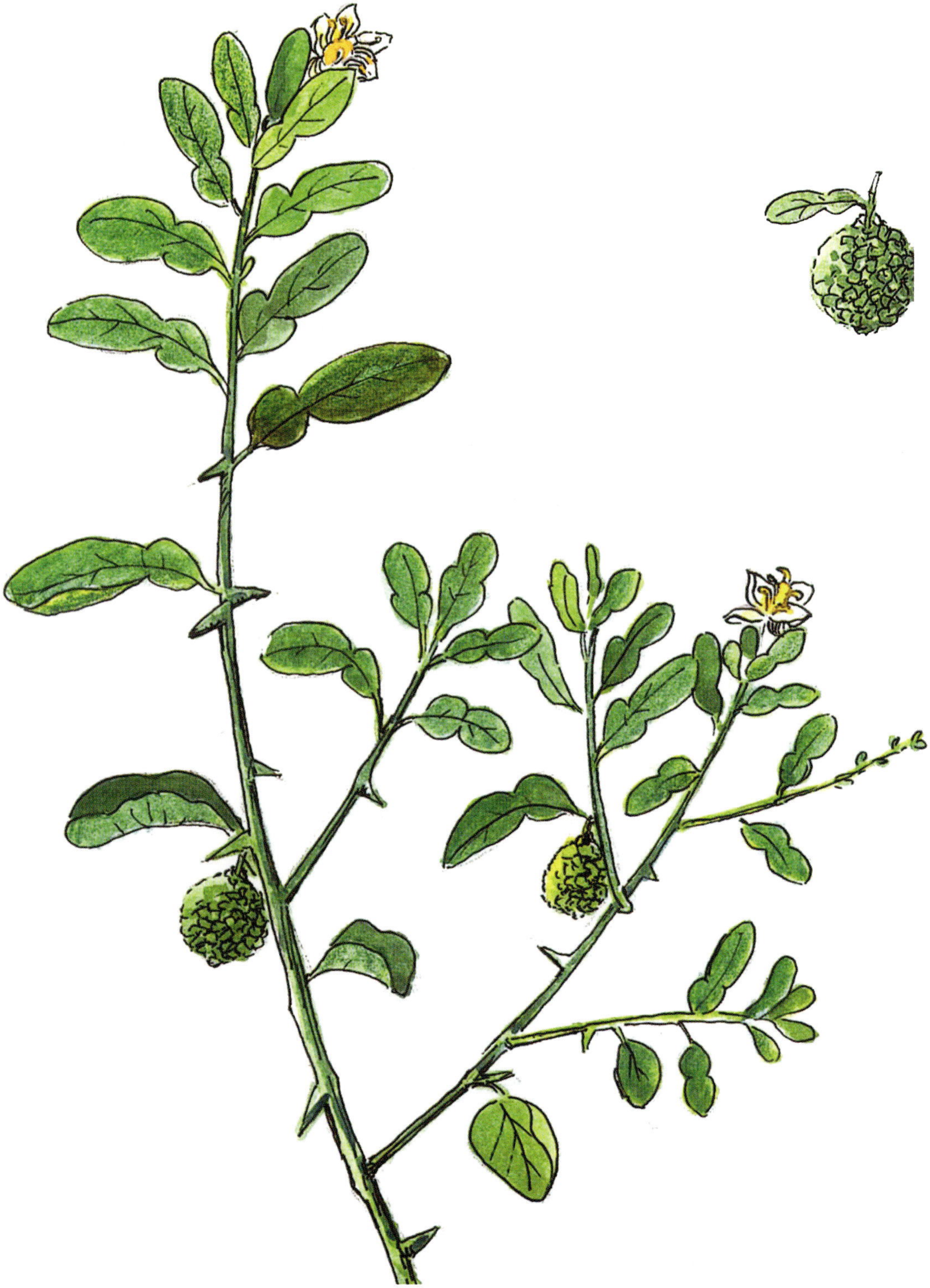

4. *Citrus sinensis (L.) Osb.*

Family: *Rutaceae*

English name: Sweet Orange

Vernacular name / Local name: *ton mak-kiang*

Name in Lao script: ຕົ້ນໝາກກ້ຽງ

Part used in saunas: leaves

Description:

A small evergreen tree with thorny branches. The leaves are ovate with wings at the base, shiny and dark green on the upper surface. Flowers are white and fragrant. The fruit is bigger than a lime, has a sweet pulp and non-bitter membranes.

Benefits:

Coughs, colds, expectorant, anorexia, stomacic, dizziness and nausea, cooling and calming.

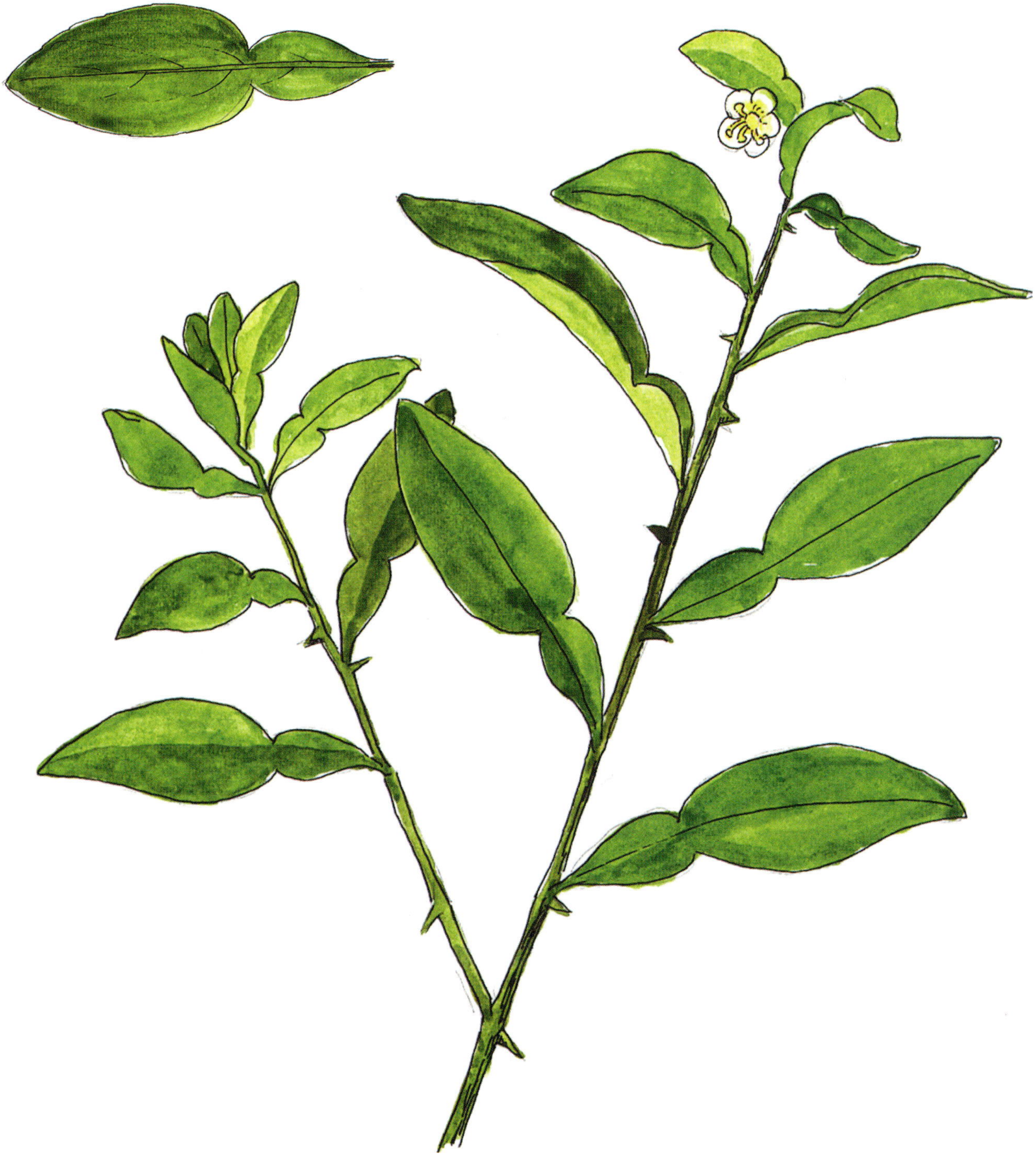

5. *Croton roxburghii N.P. Balakr.*

Family: *Euphorbiaceae*

English name: ——

Vernacular name / Local name: *ton pao nyai,ton pao*

Name in Lao script: ຕົ້ນເປົ້າໃຫຍ່, ຕົ້ນເປົ້າ

Part used in saunas: leaves

Description:

A medium shrub, 2-3 m in height. The simple leaf has a spiral arrangement and a long petiole of about 3-8 cm. The leaves are lanceolate, glabrous, serrate, green at upper surface and lighter green underneath. The size of the leaf is 4.5-9 cm wide and 8-25 cm long. Inflorescence is in the terminal spike with female and male flowers separated. The fruit is globose and up to 1 cm high.

Benefits:

Anti-toxic, cleanses the blood, prevents blood clots, bactericidal, treats nausea, helps body retain minerals, diarrhea, flatulence, vomiting.

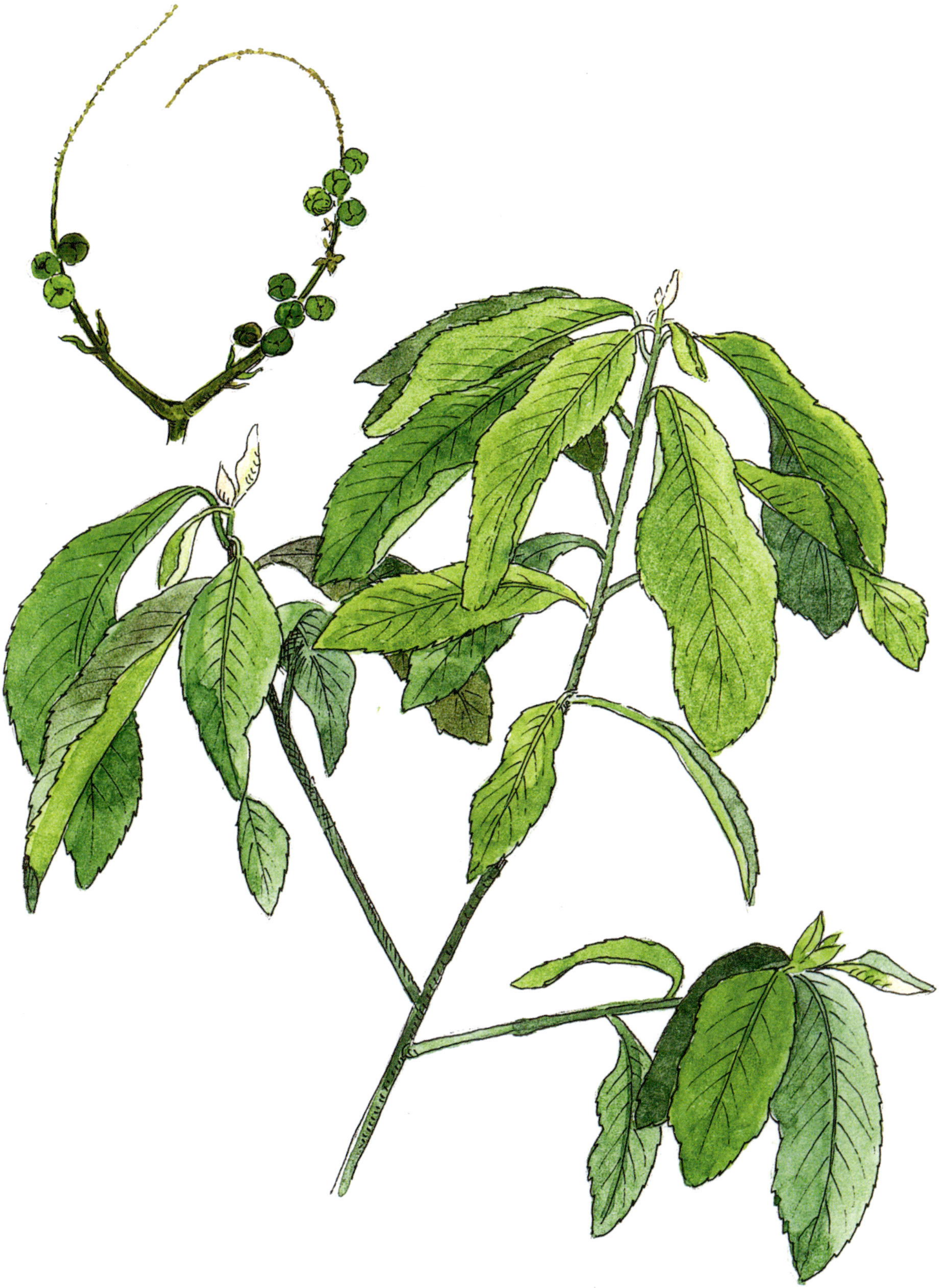

6. *Cymbopogon nardus Rendle*

Family: *Poaceae*

English name: Citronella

Vernacular name / Local name: *sii khai kheuang*

Name in Lao script: ສີໄຄເຄື່ອງ

Part used in saunas: leaves & bulb

Description:

A perennial herb with an underground rhizome. The aerial part of the plant is in two tufts, with bulb and long linear leaves, brownish-violet at maturity. There are many plants on one cluster. The tufts are longer and thicker than in Lemon Grass, *Cymbopogon citratus*, and the plant is also more highly scented than Lemon Grass.

Benefits:

Post heart attack, calming, menstrual problems, flatulance, vomiting, rheumatism, fevers, kills intestinal parasites, antiseptic, insect repellent.

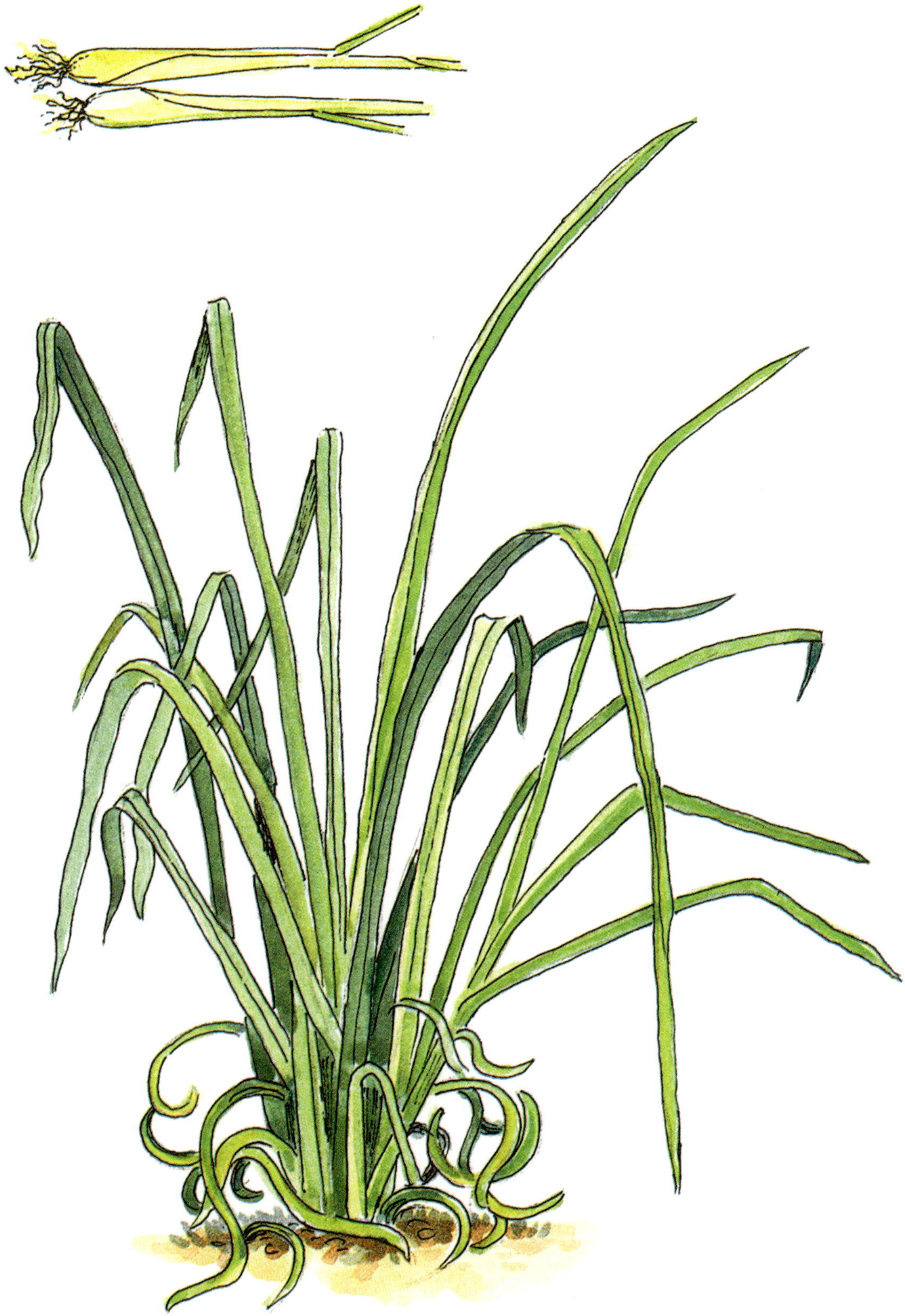

7. *Eucalyptus globulus Labill.*

Family: *Myrtaceae*

English name: Blue gum or eucalyptus

Vernacular name /Local name: *ton vik*

Name in Lao script: ຕົ້ນວິກ

Part used in saunas: leaves

Description:

A tall evergreen tree growing up to 40 m in height. The trunk is straight with a smooth pale grey bark. Young twigs are reddish-green. Leaves are aromatic, lanceolate and acute, pale green, alternate. Inflorescence is axillary, in umbels of 5 to 12, with creamy-white flowers.

Benefits:

Strong antibacterial action, wounds and skin problems, respiratory ailments and fevers, opens pores & promotes sweating.

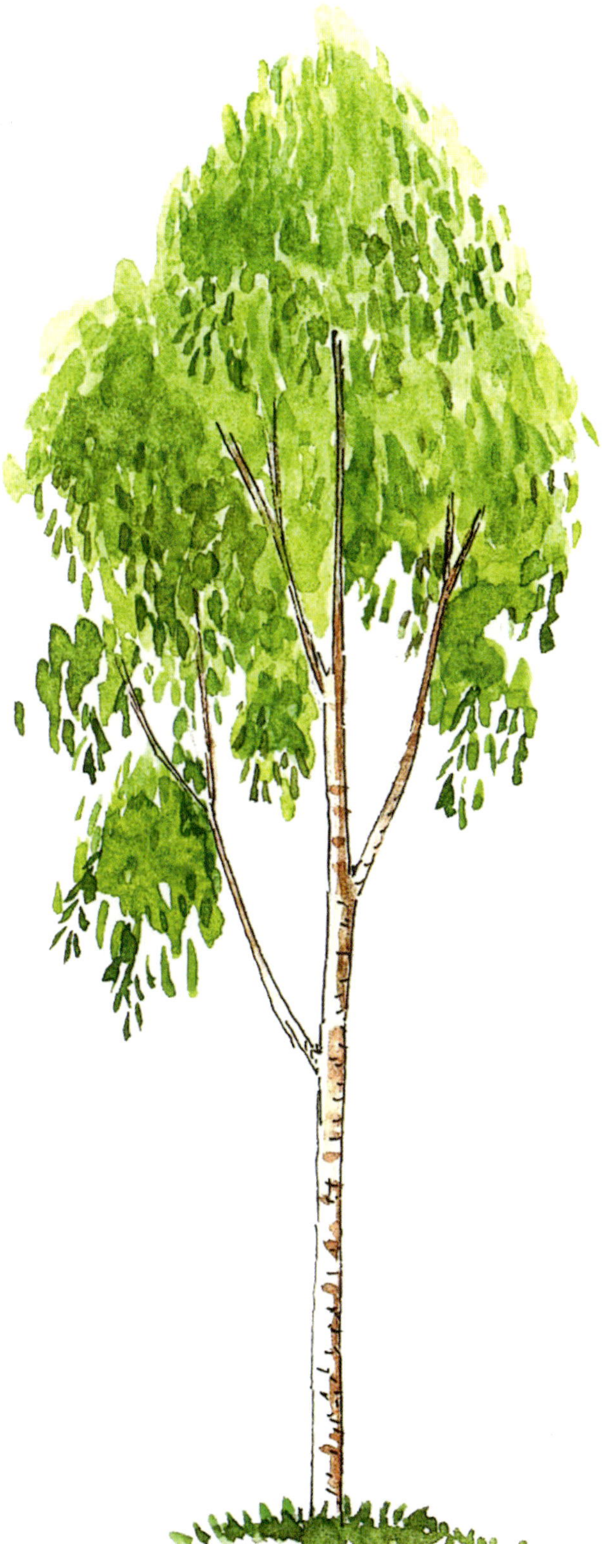

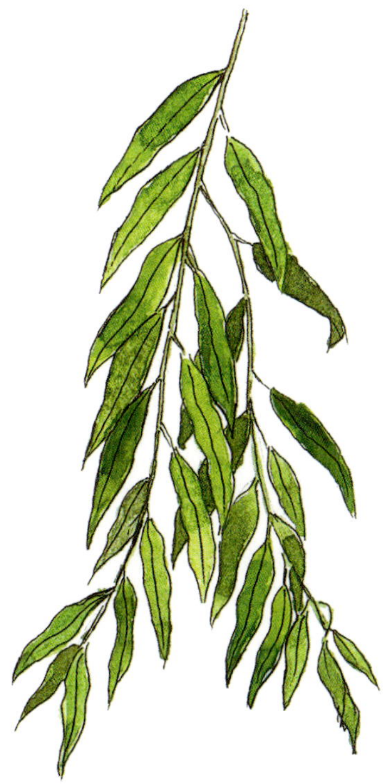

8. *Glycosmis pentaphylla Corr.*

Family: *Rutaceae*

English name: Jamaica mandarin orange

Vernacular name / Local name: *ton som seuhn*

Name in Lao script: ຕົ້ນຊົມຊື່ນ

Part used in saunas: leaves

Description:

This is a small tree, 4-6m tall. The compound leaves are imparipinnate, with a spiral arrangement. The leaflets are alternate on one petiole. The leaf has a strong smooth texture in deep green. Each leaflet is a lanceolate shape with a blade sinuate margin and is oblique at the base. The leaf is 4 to 4.5 cm wide and 8 to 10 cm long and has a slightly astringent scent. Fruits are produced in panicle form and when mature are about 1 cm in diameter and 0.8 cm in height. They are reddish brown in colour, sweet and edible. Seeds are dark brown with a hard shell.

Benefits:

Synergistic relationship with Camphor (*ton naat*), controls itchiness, assists in post-partum depression, anorexia, headaches, skin beauty.

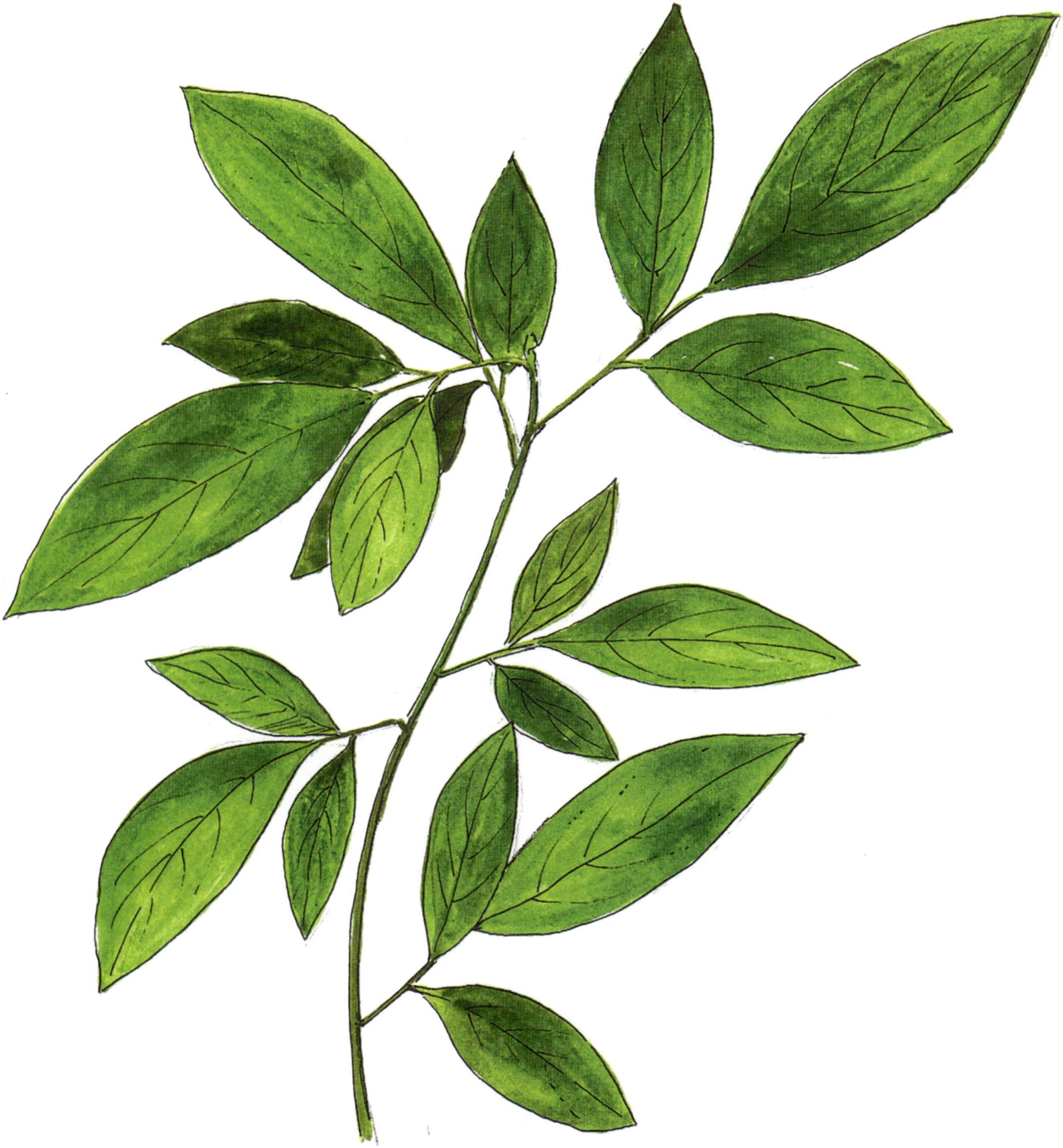

9. *Ichnocarpus frutescens (L.)W.T. Aiton*

Family: *Apocynaceae*

English name: Black creeper

Vernacular name / Local name: *kheua en ohrn*

Name in Lao script: ເຄືອເອັນອ່ອນ

Part used in saunas: Leaves and cut vine stems

Description:

A climbing vine with a long green stem of some 5-6 metres, showing internodes approximately 2-8 cm apart. The simple leaf is arranged opposite and has an elliptical shape. It is soft with a deep green upper and is whitish green underneath. Each leaf has an entire blade and apiculate apex. They are smooth and average between 2-7 cm in width and 7-15.5 cm in length. The flower is pale yellow, or creamy white, and appears in a large axillary panicle. The stem produces a milky sap. The green fruits are grouped in pairs.

Benefits:

Strengthens and maintains the nervous system, relieves paralysis, tonic.

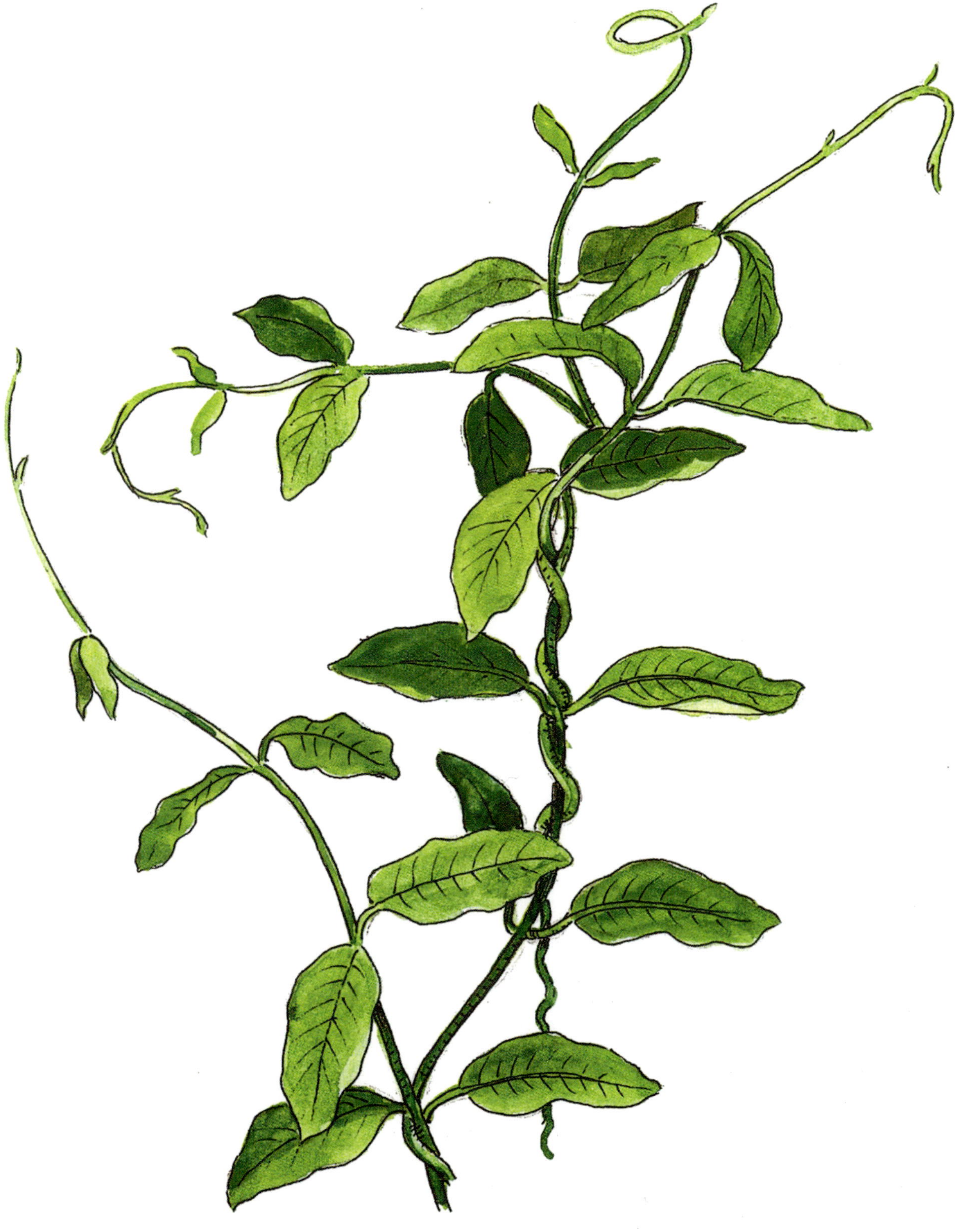

10. *Limnophila geoffrayi Bon.*

Family: *Scrophulariaceae*

English name: Bug herb

Vernacular name / Local name: *phak kha-nyaehn*

Name in Lao script: ພັກຂະແຍງ

Part used in saunas: flowers, leaves & stems

Description:

A herb, 20-30 cm tall, growing in wet or flooded rice paddy fields. It has a hairy and reddish soft stem and is lanceolate. Sessile and opposite leaves of 2.4-1.5 cm with serrate blade. Inflorescence in axillary and terminal raceme, flowers with violet corolla. The young leaves are highly fragrant.

Benefits:

Dizziness, calming, flatulance, antispasmodic.

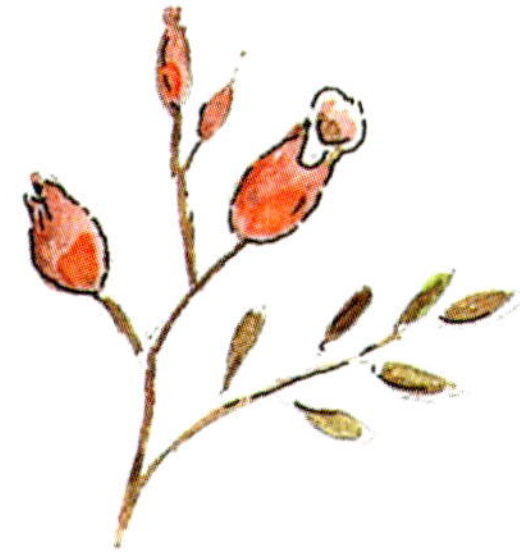

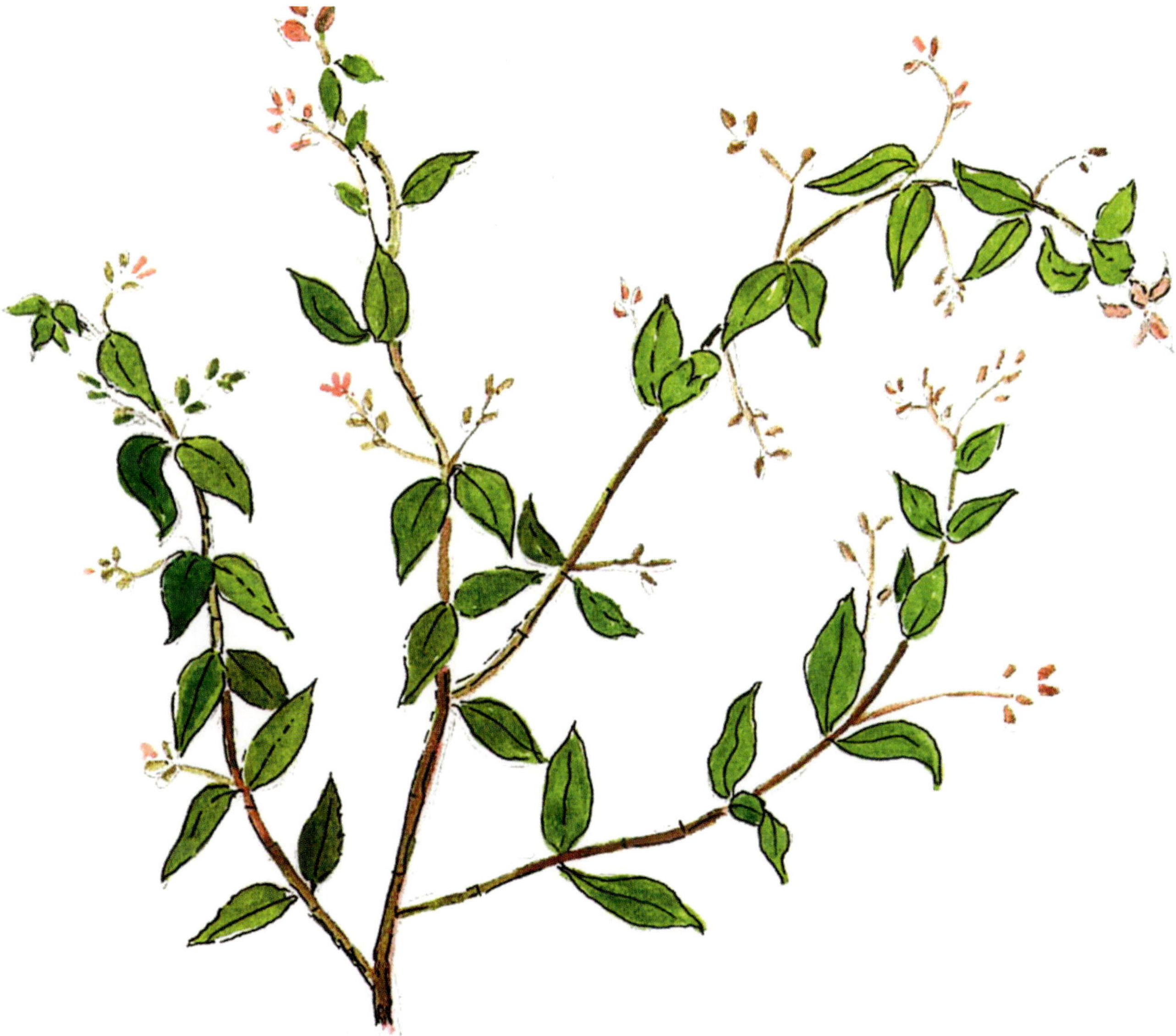

11. *Mentha arvensis Linn.*

Family: *Lamiaceae*

English name: Japanese mint

Vernacular name / Local name: *saalanat, kaalabuun*

Name in Lao script: ສາລະນາດ, ກາລະບຸນ

Part used in saunas: leaves

Description:

A ground cover plant of 10-20 cm, with erect stem end. The stem is green and tetragonal, bearing opposite leaves at node. Leaves entire, slightly pubescent, dark green at upper surface and pale green underneath. The scent of the plant is similar to that of mint.

Benefits:

Calms nervous system, respiratory ailments, anti-toxic, induces sweating, gastric upsets, headache.

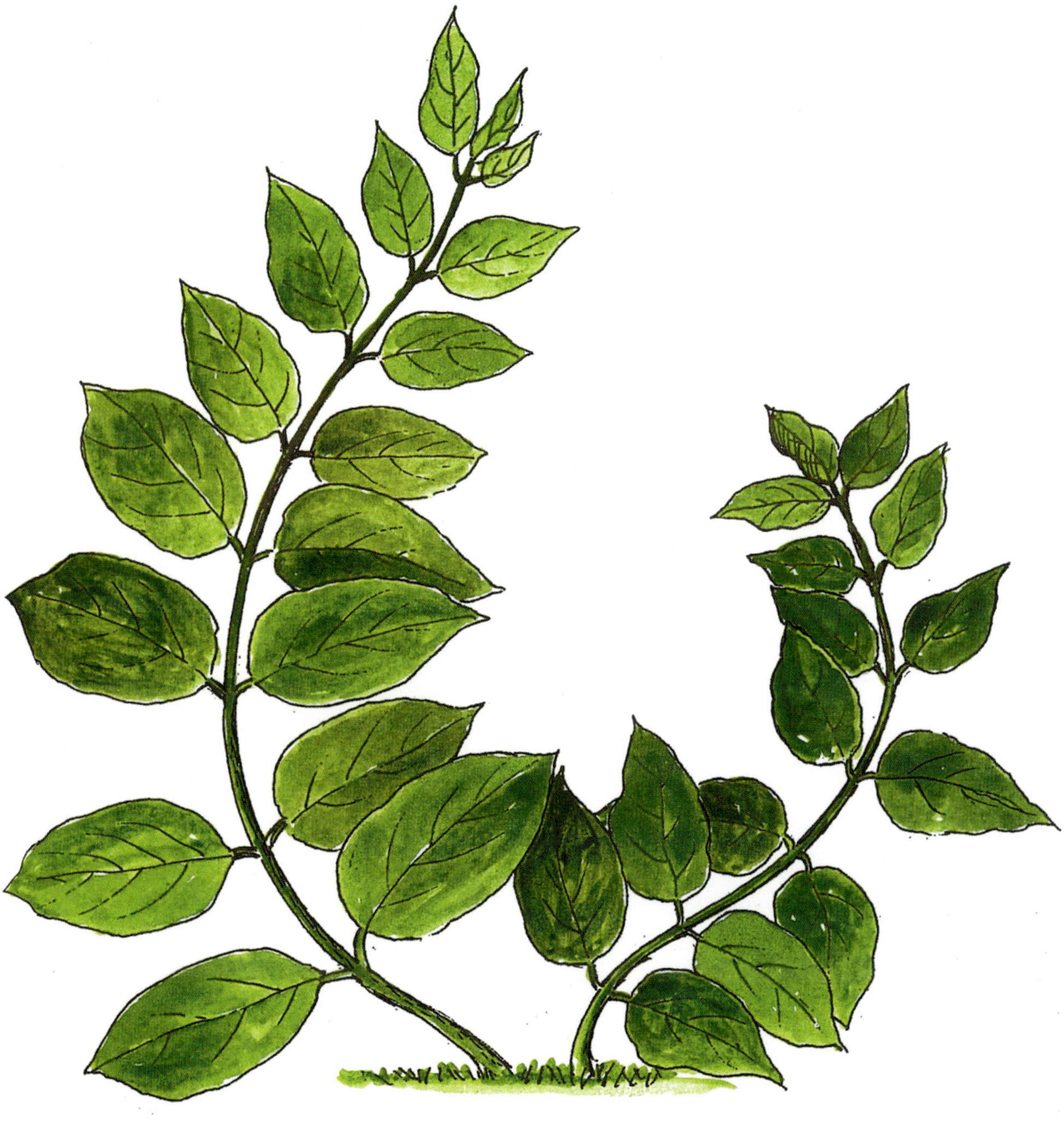

12. *Ocimum sanctum L.*

Family: *Lamiaceae*

English name: Holy Basil or Sacred Basil.

Vernacular name / Local name: *phak i-tuu laeh* or *ka-phao daehng*

Name in Lao script: ໃບຜັກອີ່ຕູ້ແລ້ ກະເຜົາແດງ

Part used in saunas: leaves

Description:

A perennial herb of about 0.80 cm in height, a reddish variety. Stem small, more or less tetragonal, strongly tomentose, pinkish-violet or pale violet. The leaves are ovate, opposite, slightly dentate, green pinkish-violet with strong scent. The flowers are pink violet and verticillated in a terminal position.

Benefits:

Lacto-stimulant, respiratory ailments, nerve tonic, muscular pain, laxative.

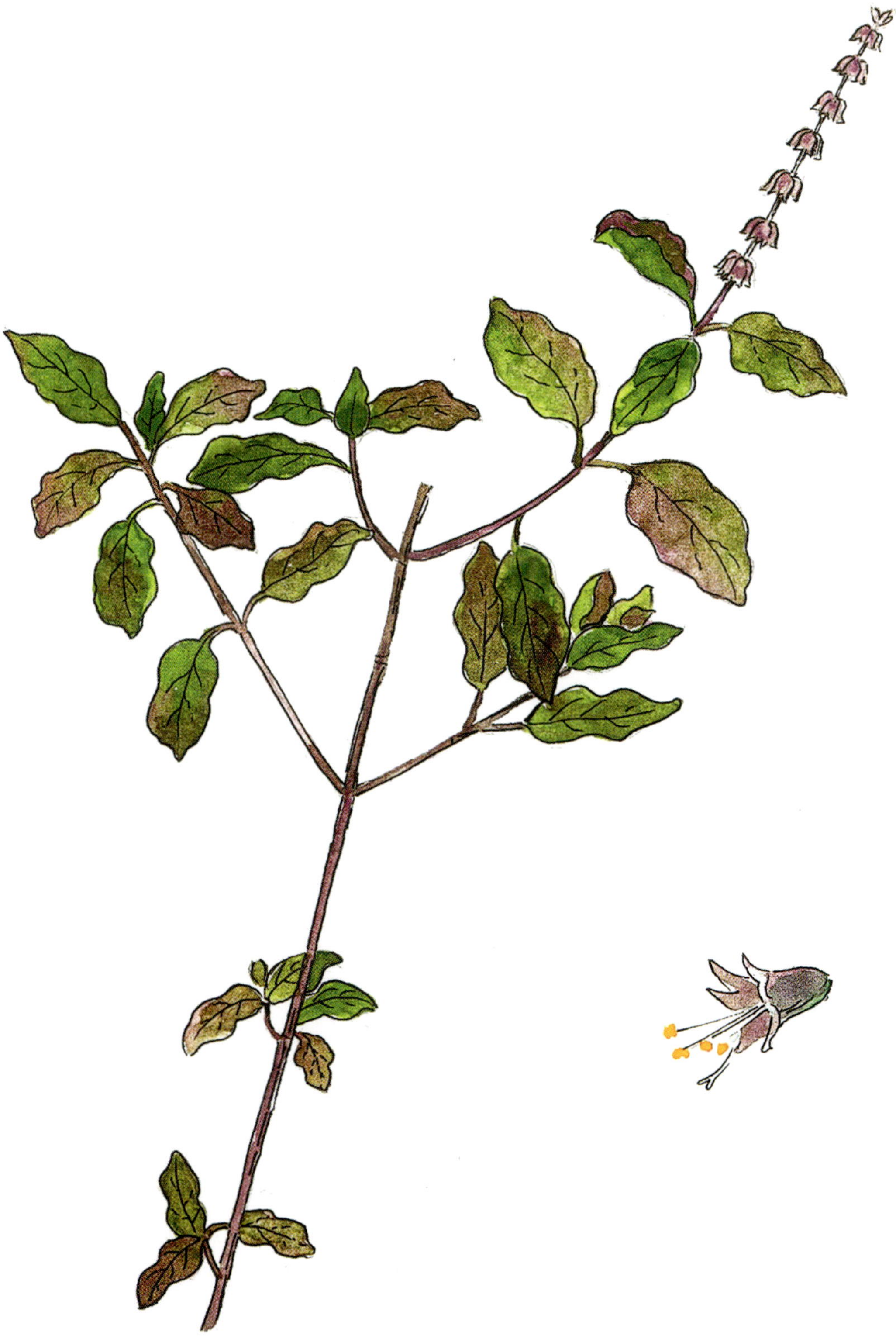

13. *Oldenlandia capitellata O.Kze*

Family: *Rubiaceae*

English name: ——

Vernacular name / Local name: *nyaa mung ka-taai*

Name in Lao script: ຫຍ້າມຸ້ງກະຕ່າຍ

Part used in saunas: leaves

Description:

A small climber, 5-8 cm long. Stem tetragonal and strongly hairy. The leaves are lanceolate and sessile, with stipules at base. Pubescent and opposite. The flowers are small, white and grouped in terminal heads.

Benefits:

Nausea, vomiting, dizziness, flatulence.

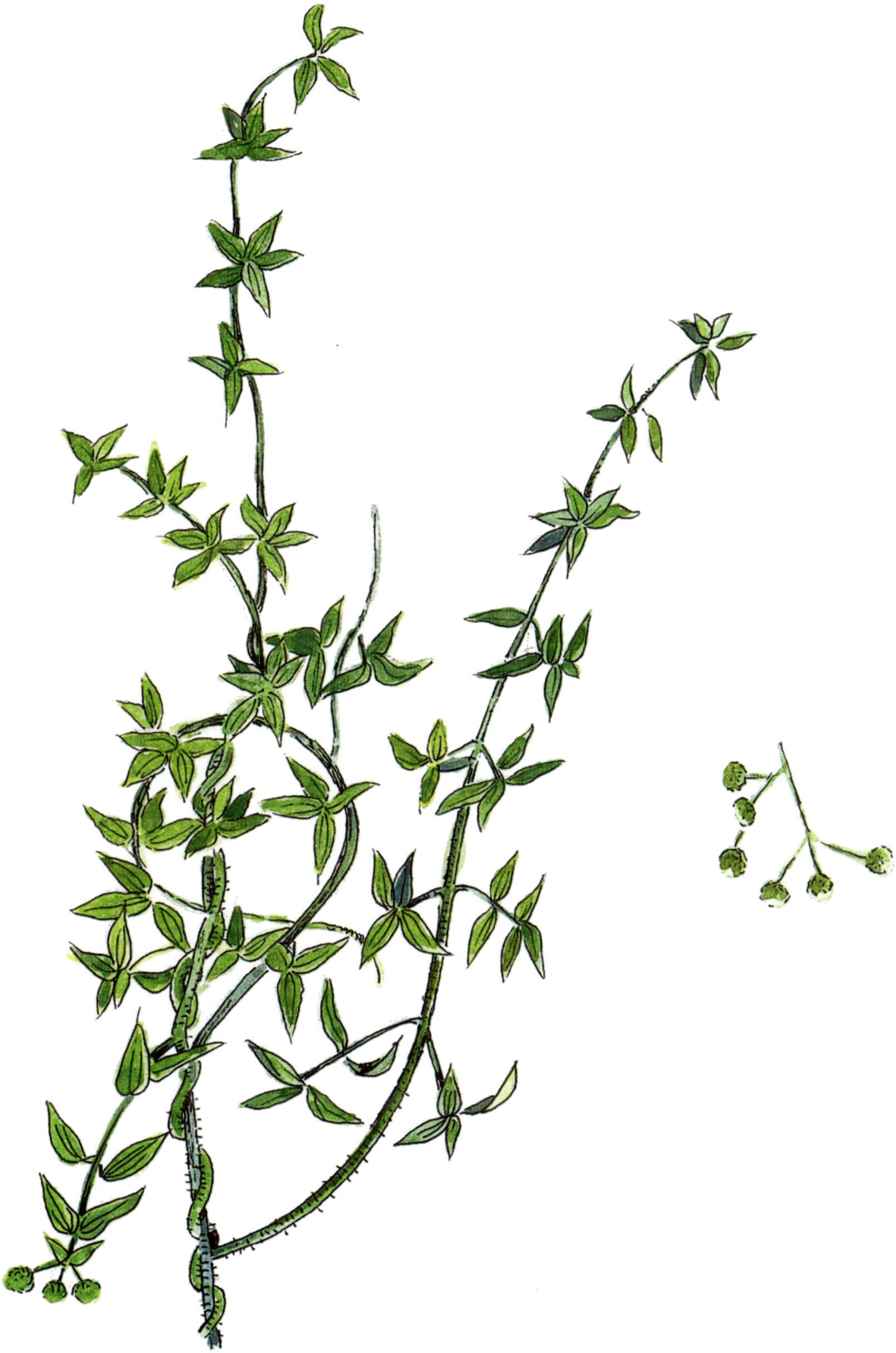

14. *Tamarindus indica Linn*

Family: *Ceasalpiniaceae*

English name: Tamarind

Vernacular name / Local name: *ton mak-khaam som*

Name in Lao script: ຕົ້ນໝາກຂາມສົ້ມ

Part used in saunas: leaves & fruit

Description:

A tall tree 15-25 m tall. The leaves are pinnate and arranged alternately, with up to 12 pairs of leaflets. The inflorescence in axillary and terminal raceme. The flowers are pale yellow. Fruit appears in an oblong pod, often curved; pulp is brown when ripe and sour. Young leaves, fruits, pulp (ripe and unripe) are used in cooking as well.

Benefits:

Fruit pulp can be applied before entering sauna to heal sores and wounds; it prevents dry cracking skin. The leaves and unripe fruits are boiled and the waters are used for women to bathe in after child birth, to reduce swelling and promote healing. Also used to cure coughs and reduce mucus. Rheumatism, cough and phlegm, sores and wounds, conjunctivitis, constipation, calming.

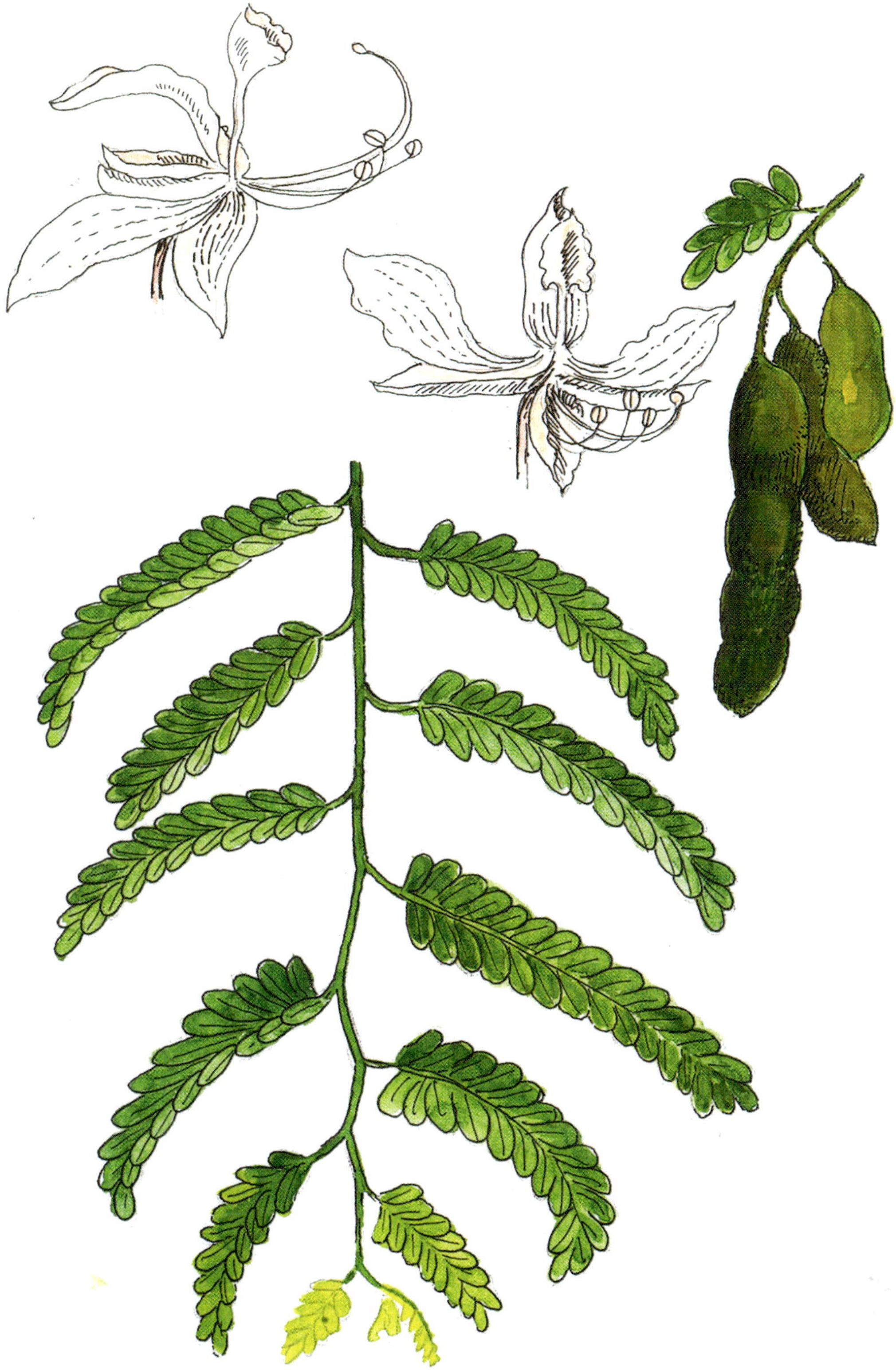

15. *Vitex trifolia L*

Family: *Verbenaceae*

English name: Indian wild pepper

Vernacular name / Local name: *phi-seua noi*

Name in Lao script: ພີເສືອນ້ອຍ

Part used in saunas: leaves

Description:

This is a medium sized tree standing 3-6 m tall. The leaves are trifoliate and opposite. The central leaflet, the largest one, is obovate with the upper a medium green and underneath a silver/white color. The width of each leaflet is between 2-2.8 cm and is 5.5-6.5 cm in length. A simple leaf is sometimes present especially at base of the branch.

Benefits:

These strongly scented leaves are frequently used in the sauna for cooling the body, for respiratory problems and as a synergistic mix with other plants. The leaves are used along with Camphor (*Ton Naad*) to reduce swelling eg - after childbirth, for rheumatism, wounds, fever, cough & mucus, diuretic.

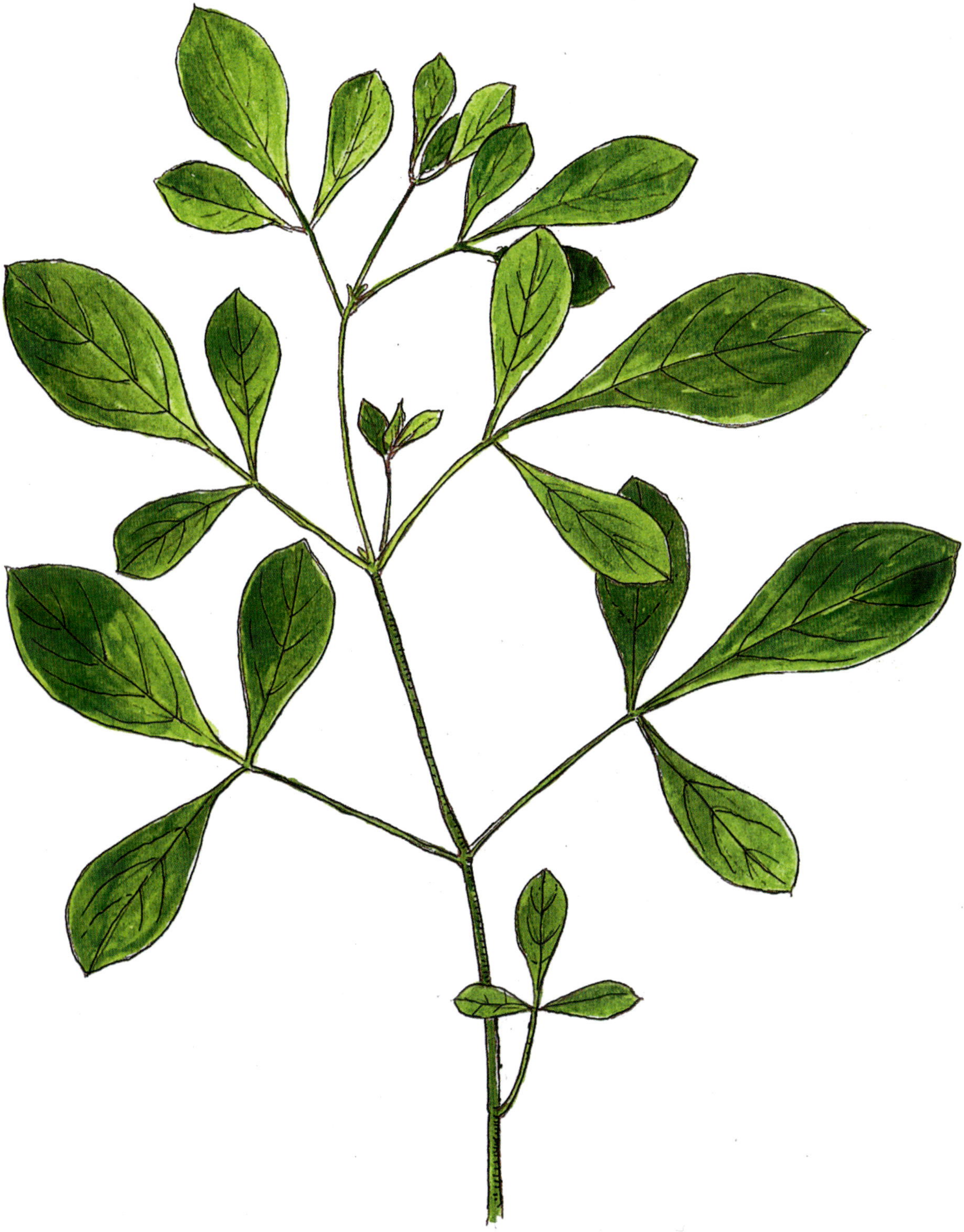

II. OCCASIONALLY USED:

16. *Citrus aurantifolia (Christm. & Pang) Swing.*

Family: *Rutaceae*

English name: Lime tree

Vernacular name / Local name: *ton mak-naao*

Name in Lao script: ຕົ້ນໝາກນາວ

Part used in saunas: leaves

Description:

A shrub 2-4 m in height. with young thorny twigs. The leaves are simple, alternate, ovate, slightly acute, rounded at the base, serrate and punctate. The petiole bears a small wing. The flowers are small, white and grouped by two and three in an axillary position. The fruit is globose with a shiny skin. Both leaves and fruit are sweet-smelling.

Benefits:

Sedative, fever, nausea, dizziness, expectorant, asthma, improves circulation, colds, acne, infections, detoxification, anti-inflammatory, improves menstruation, stimulates sweating

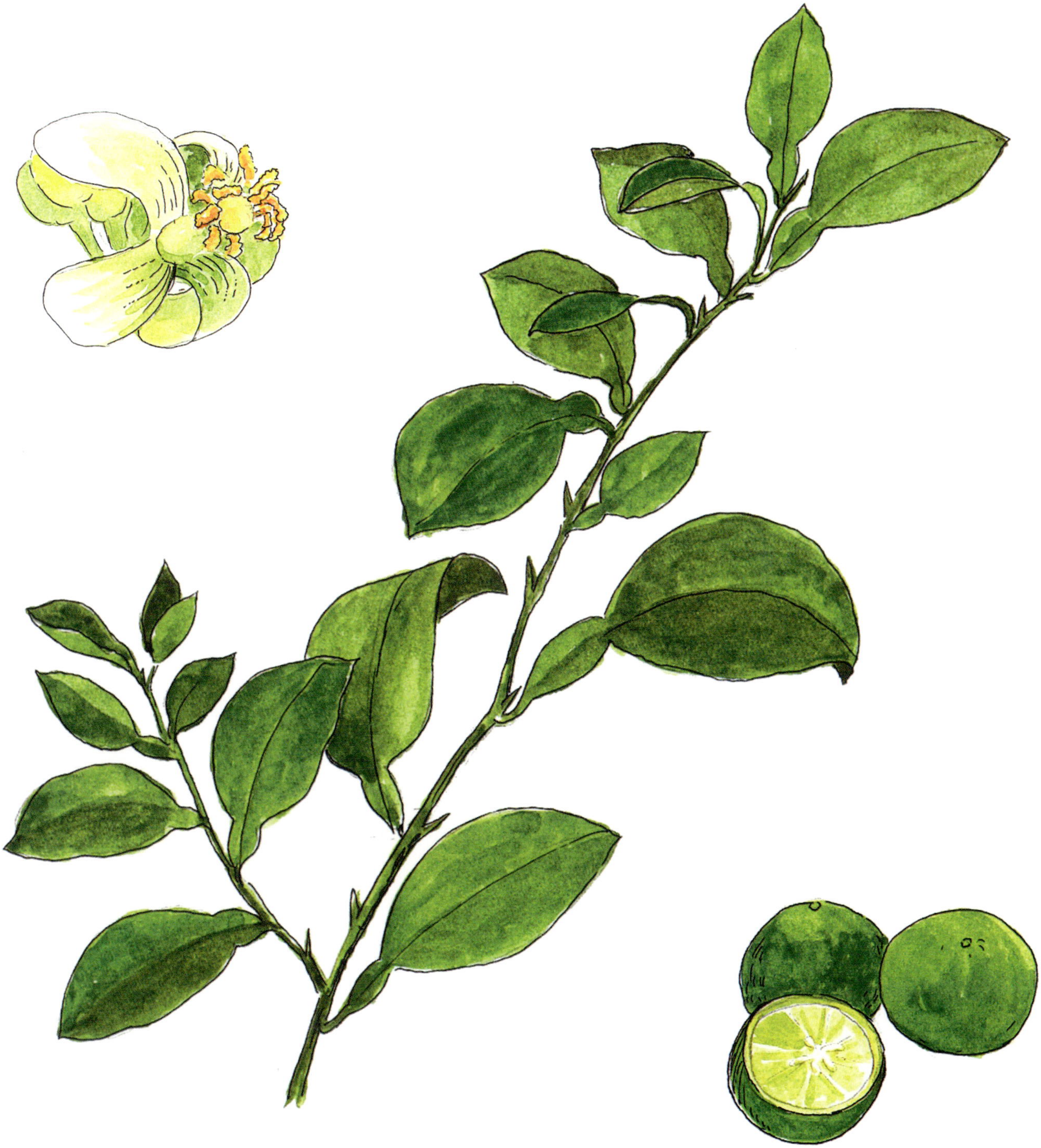

17. *Coleus ambonicus Lour.*

Family: *Lamiaceae*

English name: Indian borage

Vernacular name / Local name: *huu seua*

Name in Lao script: ຫູເສືອ

Part used in saunas: leaves

Description:

A perennial herbaceous plant, 30-50 cm in height. Soft stemed and strongly tomentose. The leaves are thick and as wide as they are long at about 5 cm. They are ovate, crenate, hirsute and arranged opposite. The whole plant is highly scented.

Benefits:

Overheating especially in children, treats wounds, headaches, coughs, stomach ailments.

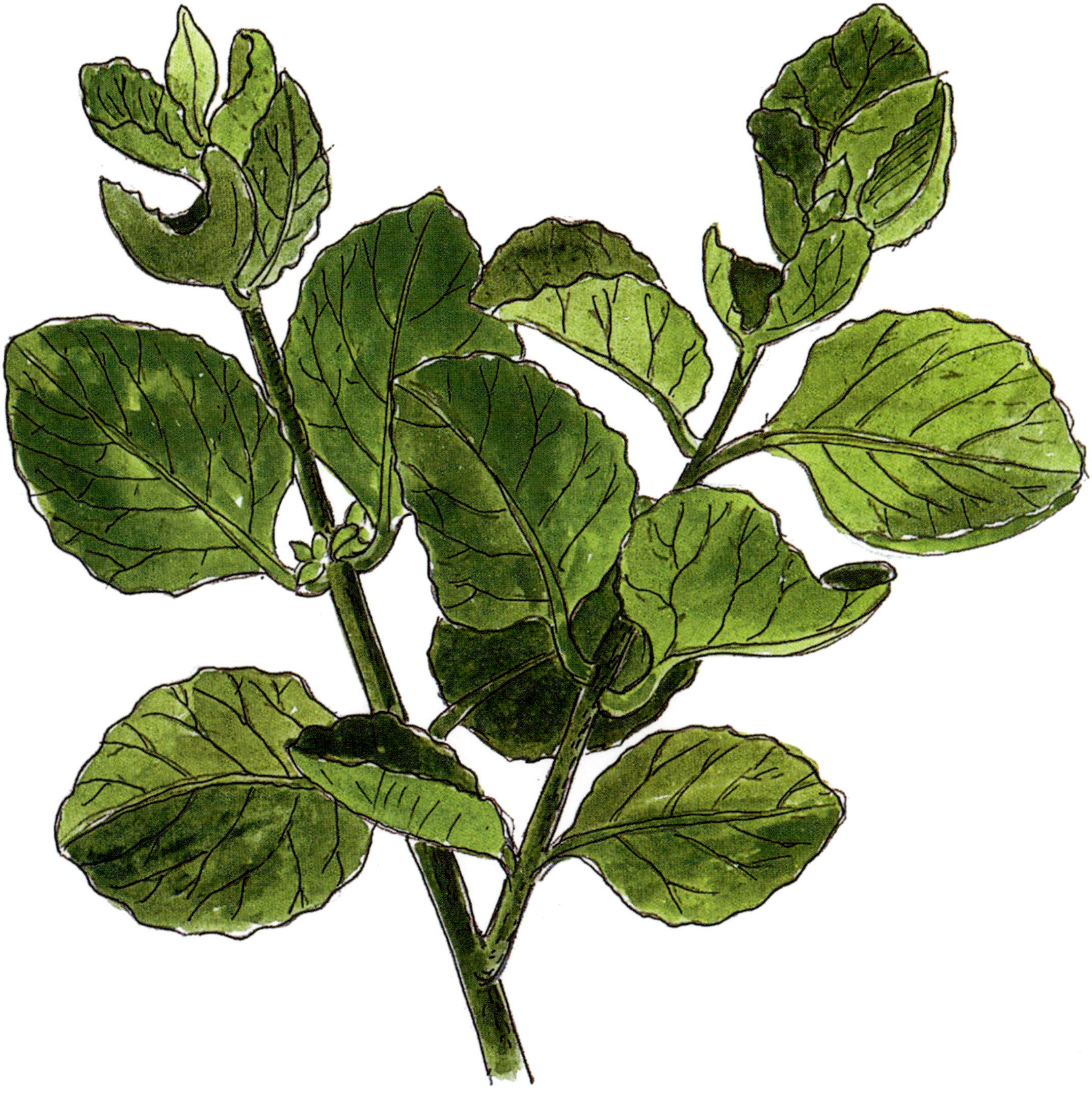

18. *Conyza aurita L.f.*

Family: *Asteraceae*

English name: ——

Vernacular name / Local name: *naat nao*

Name in Lao script: ໜາດເໜົ່າ

Part used in saunas: leaves

Description:

A herbaceous plant of 50-80 cm, growing wild in unused garden spaces. The stem is stiff; the leaves sessile, obovate, biserrate and arranged alternately. Leaf excrescence on a long stem. Inflorescence the compound of a big head panicle in terminal position. Flowers violet or pale yellow when young. The whole silvery, velutinous plant is highly fragrant..

Benefits:

Excellent for post-partum healing and the relief of headaches.

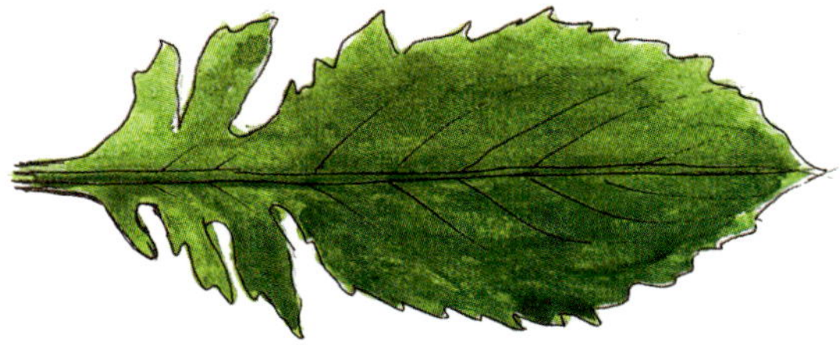

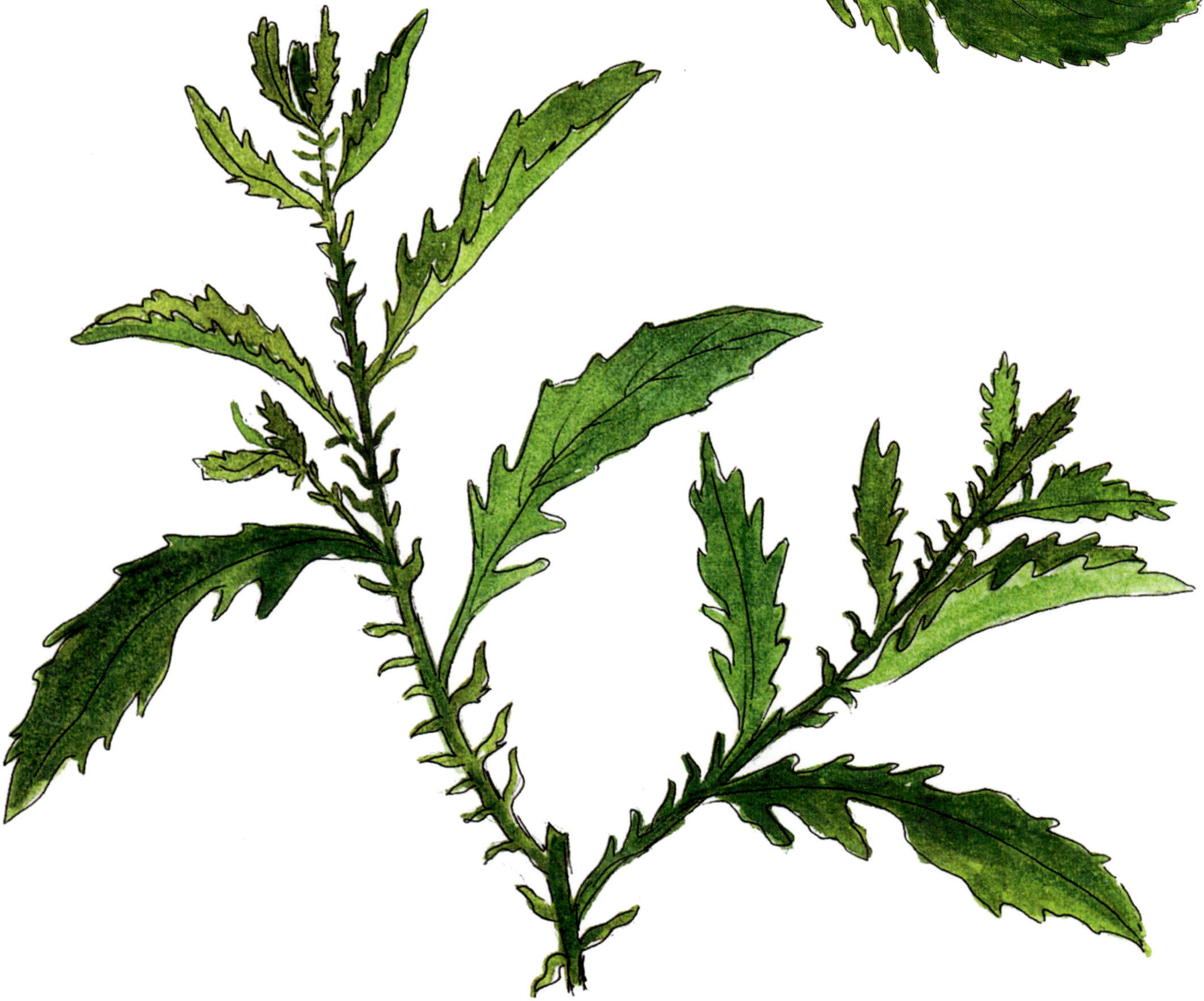

19. *Micromelum minutum (Forst.f.) Wight & Arn.*

Family: *Rutaceae*

English name: Lime berry / Orange berry / Butterfly tree

Vernacular name / Local name: *ton sa-mat*

Name in Lao script: ຕົ້ນສະມັດ

Part used in saunas: leaves

Description:

A small tree, 5 m in height with pubescent young twigs. The leaves are arranged in alternate spiral compound leaflets. An individual leaflet oblique at base has a punctuate blade underneath and on the margin. The width of each leaf is about 2.5-3 cm and 3-11 cm long. The inflorescence is in a terminal panicle with numerous small creamy-white flowers. The fruits have fine hair and when mature are yellow-red in colour. They have an astringent smell with one green seed in each fruit measuring about 0.5x 0.8 cm.

Benefits:

In the sauna, leaves are used as a stimulant. The roots can also be used in compresses for boils and skin ulcers, tightens sagging flesh, assists in post-partum healing.

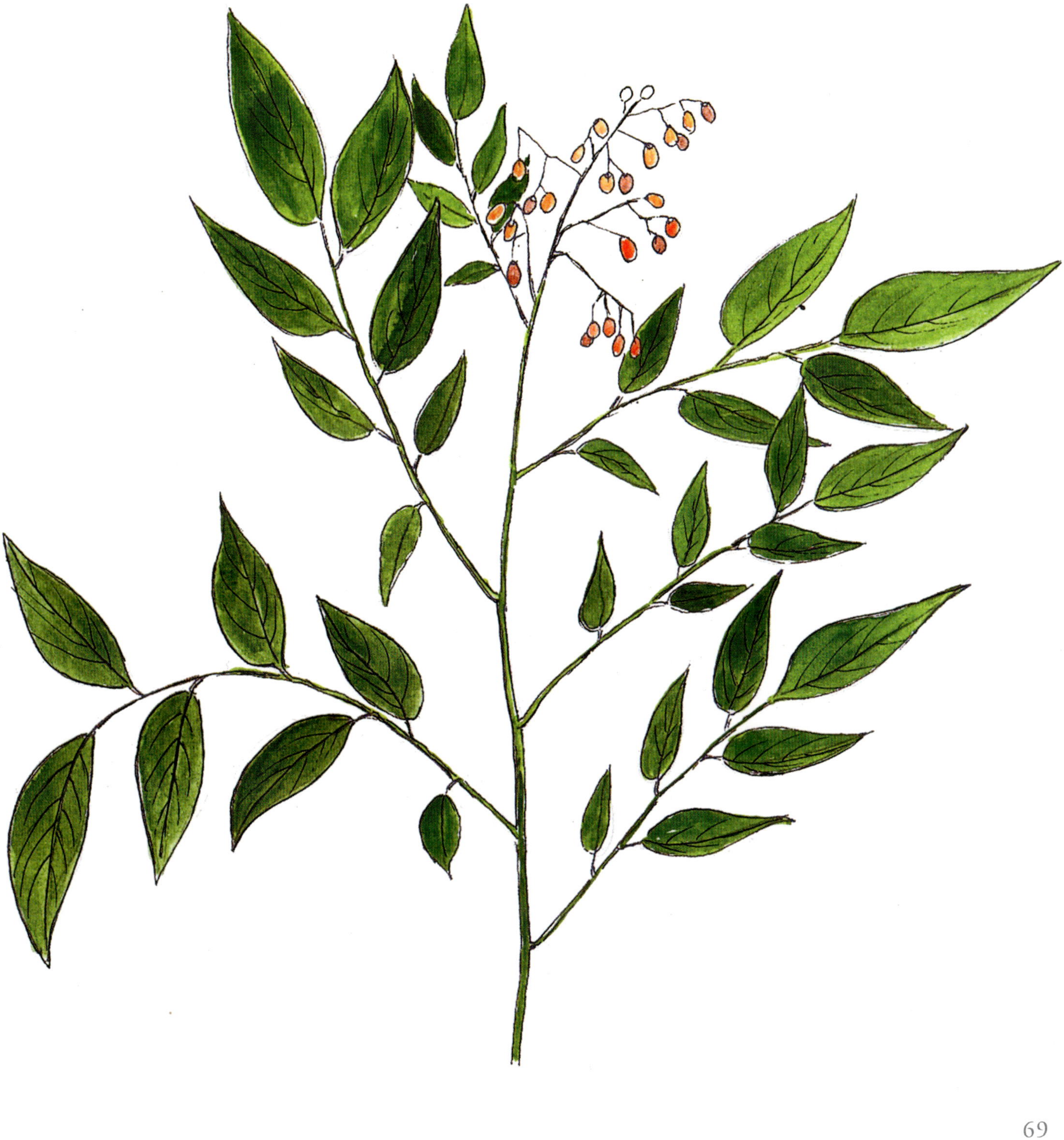

20. *Ocimum gratissimum Linn.*

Family: *Lamiaceae*

English name: Hairy Basil

Vernacular name / Local name: *phak i-tuu nyai*

Name in Lao script: ພັກອີ່ຕູ່ໃຫຍ່

Part used in saunas: leaves

Description:

A small shrub 1-2 m in height. The leaves are 4-7 cm wide and 8-14 cm long, ovate, strongly dentate and opposite with long petioles of up to 2 cm long. The flowers are verticillated, in a terminal position, with yellowish white corolla and a purplish green upper lip.

Benefits:

Antispasmodic, antidepressant, nerve tonic, warming, restorative, treats stomach ailments.

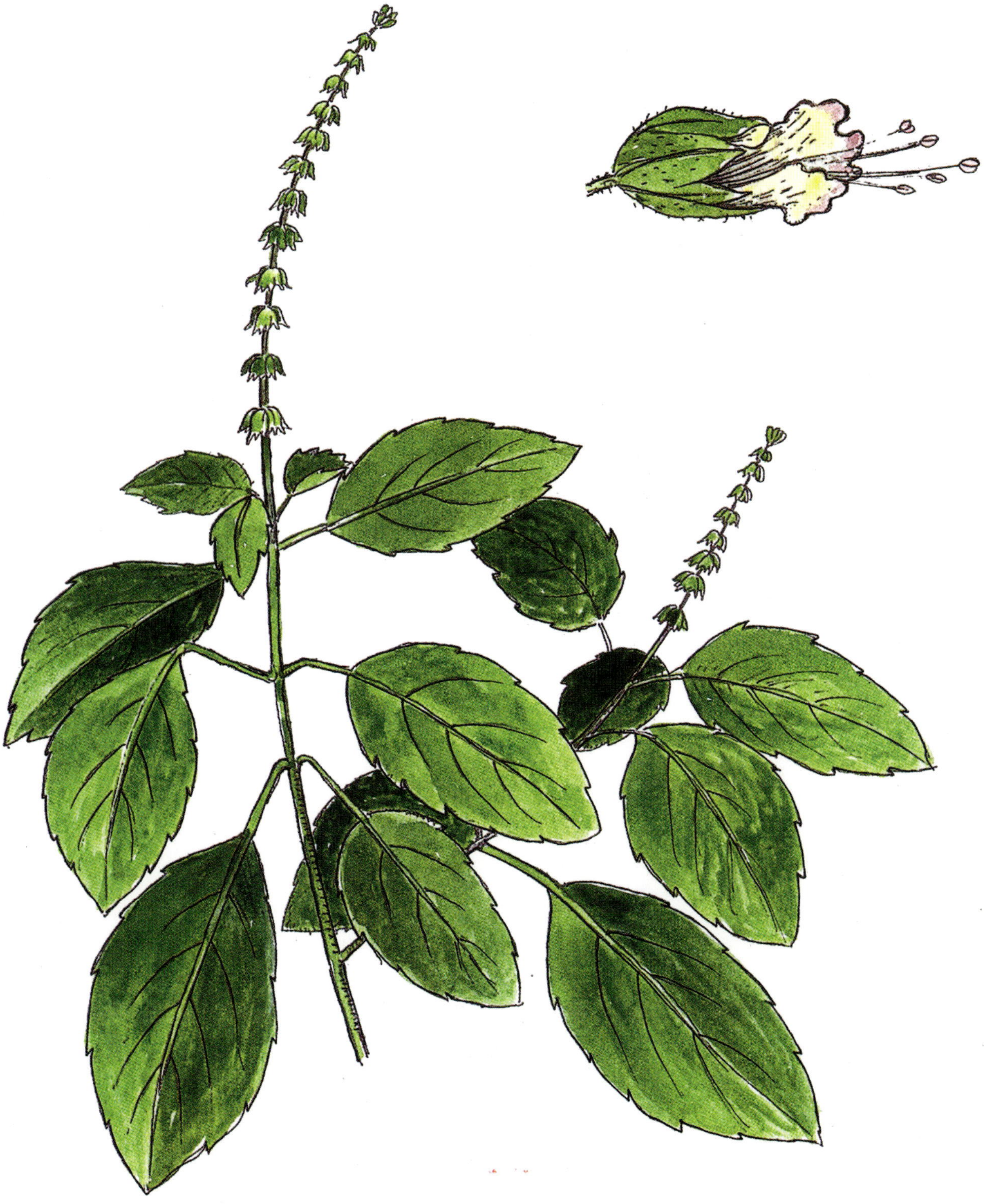

21. *Ocimum sanctum L.*

Family: *Lamiaceae*

English name: White Holy Basil or Sacred Basil

Vernacular name / Local name: *phak i-tuu khiao noi* or *ka-phao khaao*

Name in Lao script: ພັກອີ່ຕູ່ຂຽວນ້ອຍ, ກະເຜົາຂາວ

Part used in saunas: leaves

Description:

A white variety of *Ocimum sanctum* that differs from the reddish variety. The leaves and twigs are green, the stem brown and the flowers whitish-green. The young leaves of the white variety are more often used in cooking than the reddish variety.

Benefits:

Sedative and antidepressant, nerve tonic, fever, lacto-stimulant, muscular and diuretic, induces menstruation, laxative.

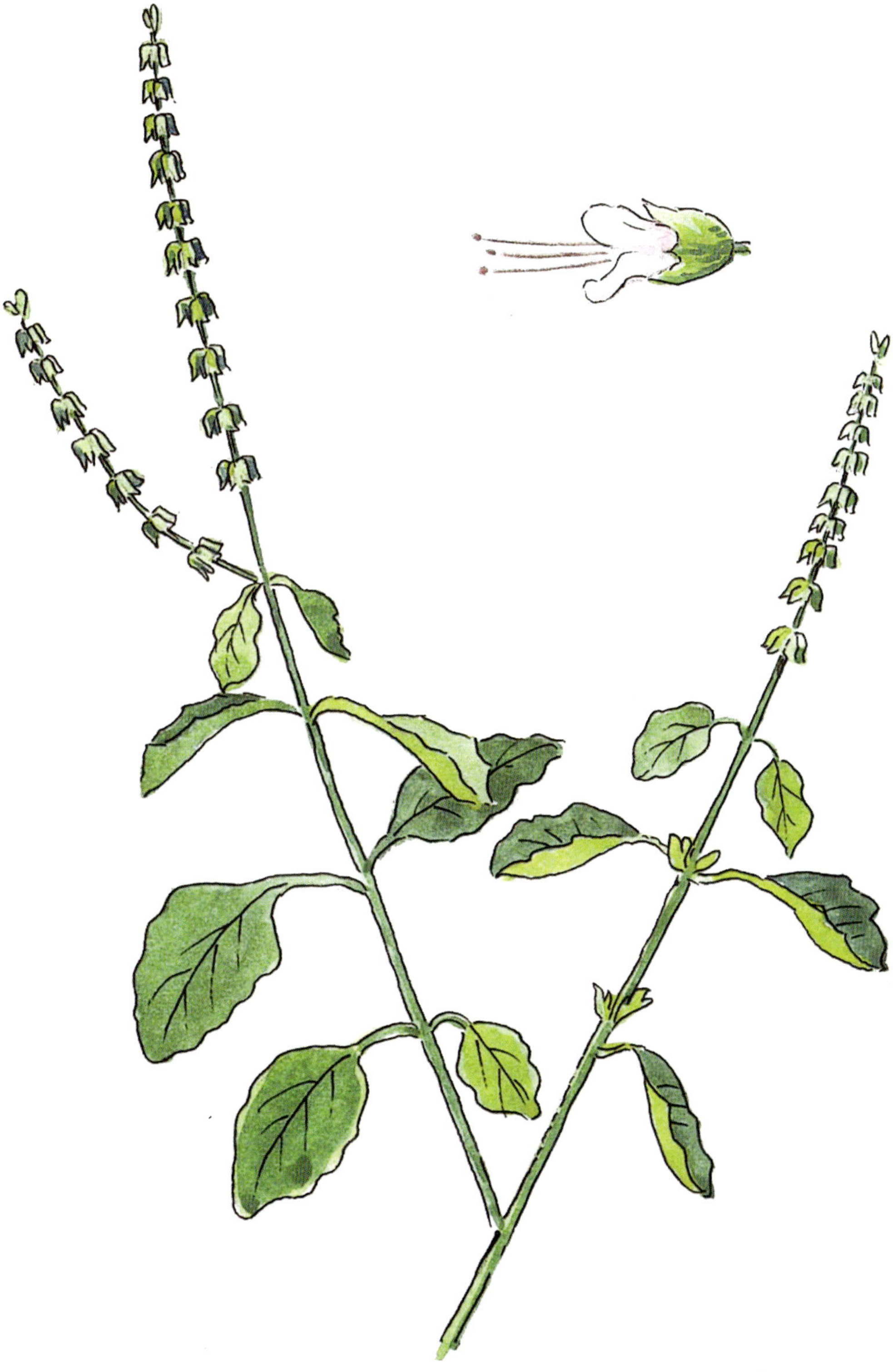

22. *Zingiber purureum Rosc.*

Family: *Zingiberaceae*

English name: Chinese ginger

Vernacular name / Local name: *vaan phai*

Name in Lao script: ຫວານໄພ

Part used in saunas: stems, leaves & chopped rhizome

Description:

A plant with a grass-like character that reaches a height of 0.5-1.5 metres. The stem is soft, green and bearing alternate dark green leaves. Flowers are pale yellow and grouped in a dense spike. They are encased in a involucre of green bracts that envelop half of the flowers. The plant dies off when the rhizome is mature and will grow back again during the next rainy season.

Benefits:

Fainting, indigestion, flatulence, fevers & stomach problems.

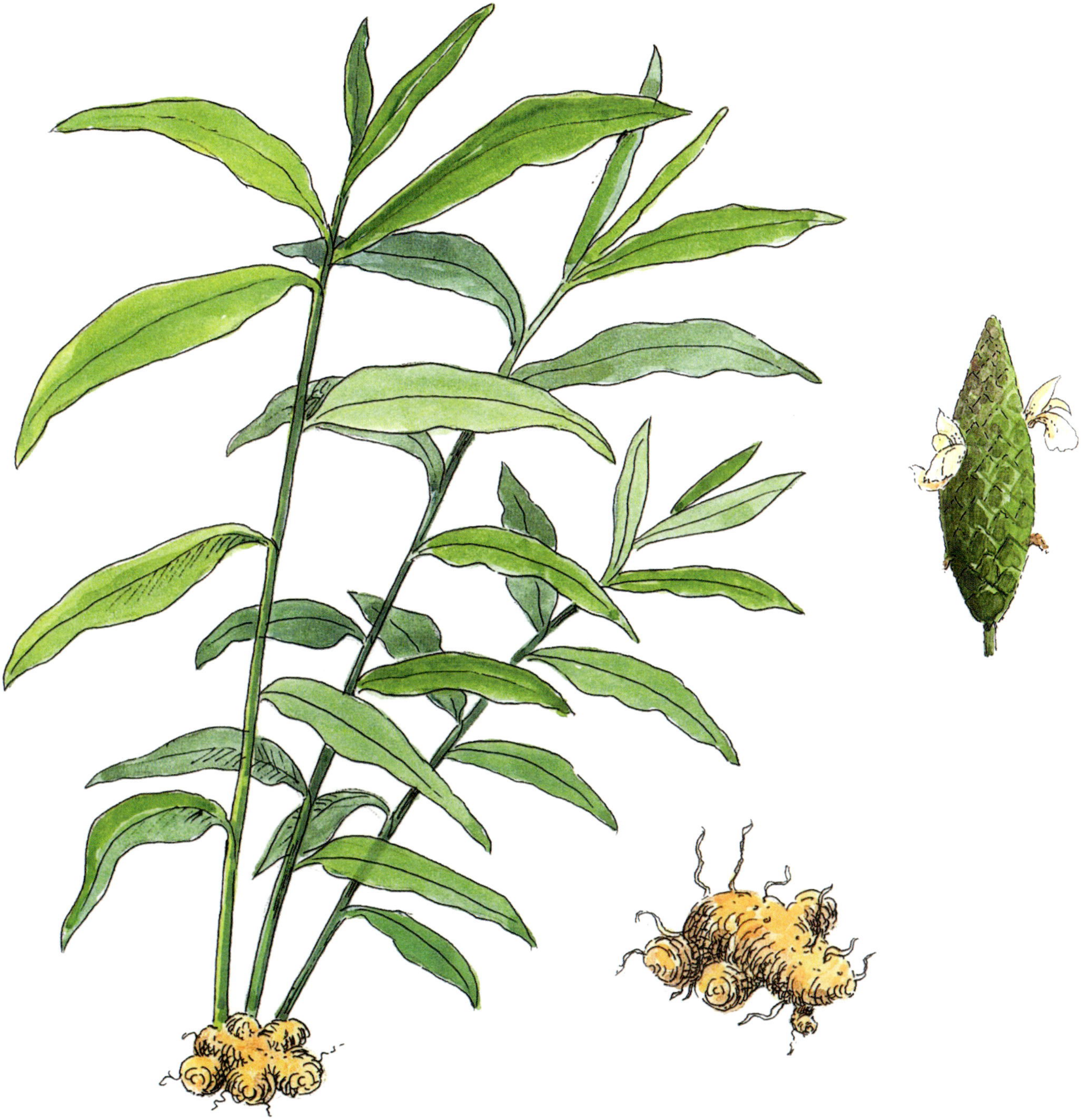

III. USED FOR SPECIAL AILMENTS :

23. *Alstonia scholaris (L.) R.Br.*

Family: *Apocynaceae*

English name: Devil tree

Vernacular name / Local name: *ton tiin pet*

Name in Lao script: ຕົ້ນຕີນເປັດ

Part used in saunas: leaves

Description:

A tree 12-20 m high, strongly milky. It's leaves are oblanceolate, acuminate and arranged in whorls of 5 to 6. Flowers are white in a dense cluster and fruits are grouped in pairs, in long and slender cylindrical follicles.

Benefits:

Prevents bone loss, indigestion, flatulence, stomach ailments, general tonic, treats malaria, fever, skin diseases, bactericidal.

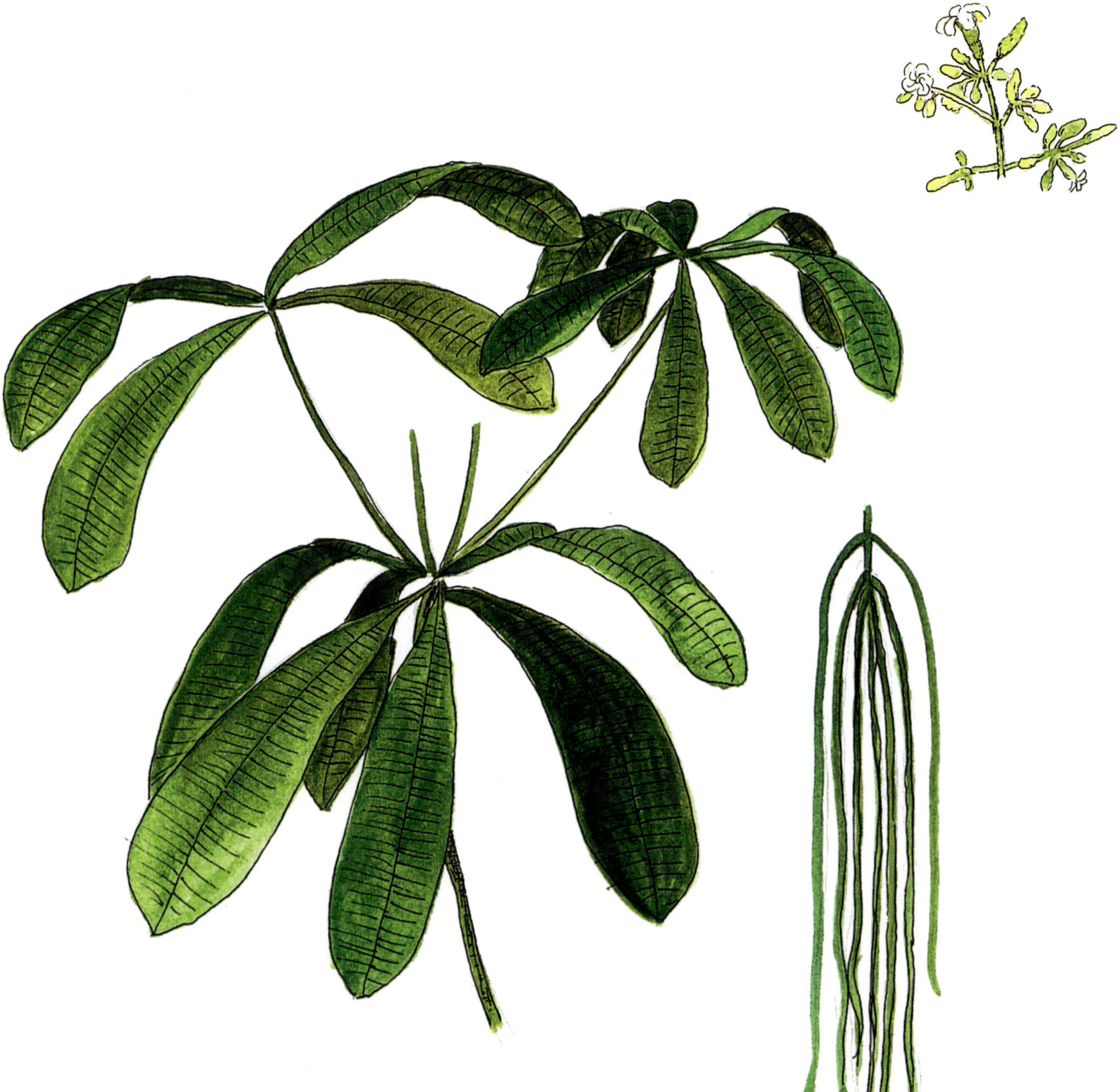

24. *Averrhoa carambola Linn.*

Family: *Oxalidaceae*

English name: Star fruit

Vernacular name / Local name: *ton mak-feuang*

Name in Lao script: ຕົ້ນໝາກເຟືອງ

Part used in saunas: leaves

Description:

A medium sized tree of 5-6 m. Leaves pinnate and alternate with 2-11 lanceolate leaflets, 2-3.5 in wide and 3-9 cm long. Petiole is swollen at base. Inflorescence is in axillary panicle and flower reddish-purple. The fruit is a berry, approximately 5-10 cm long, light green to yellow on maturing. The shape is like a star when sliced. Taste is sour.

Benefits:

Chickenpox, ringworm, headache, fever, chills, intestinal disorders.

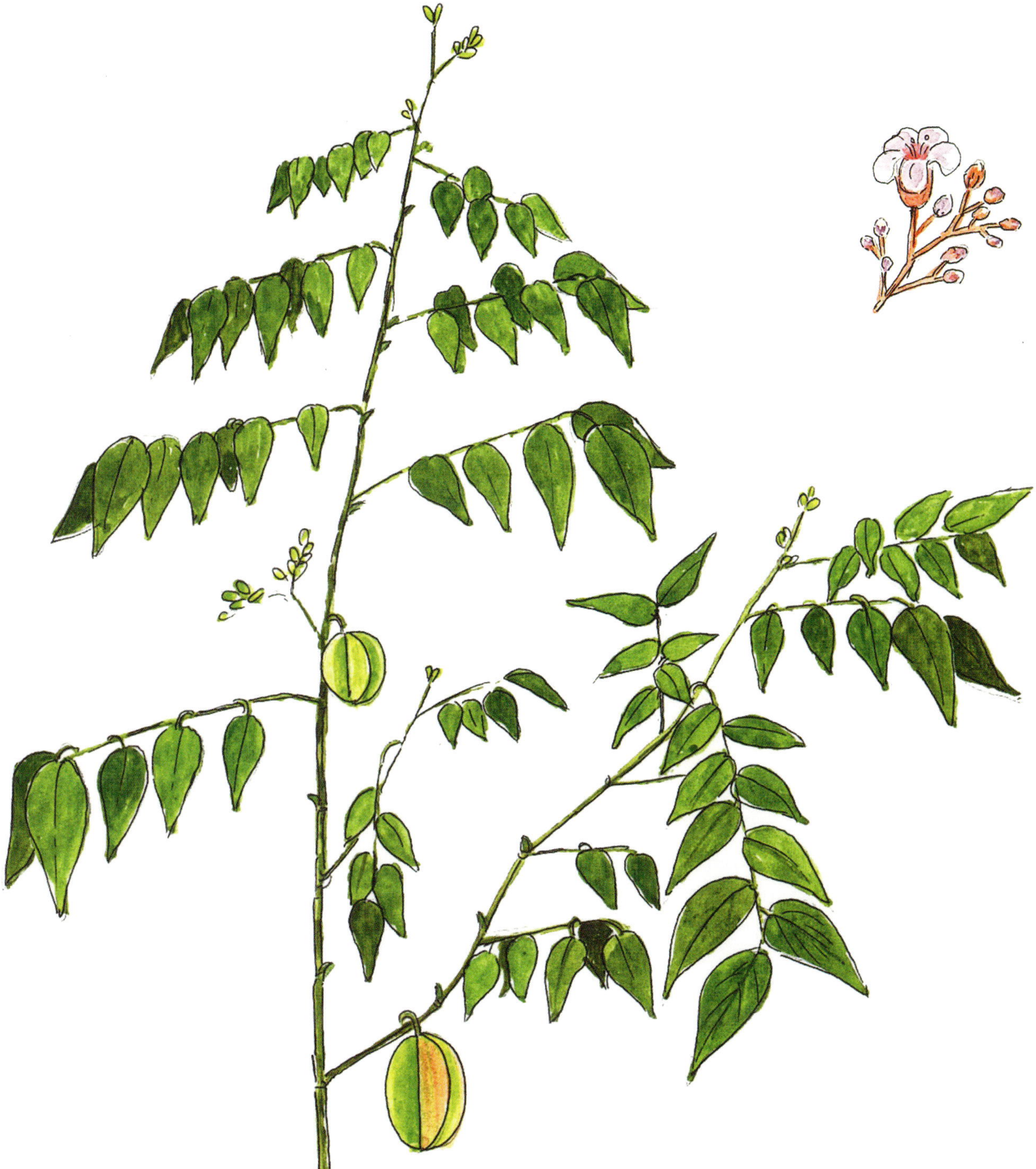

25. *Cinnamomum cassia (Nees) Nees & Eberh.*

Family: *Lauraceae*

English name: Chinese cassia

Vernacular name / Local name: *ton juang* or *saa juang*

Name in Lao script: ຕົ້ນຈວງ

Part used in saunas: leaves

Description:

A tree up to 30 m high. Bark grayish-brown. Leaves are simple, elliptic-oblong or lanceolate-oblong, dark green, thick and opposite, measuring 3-4 cm x 8-15 cm with 3 veins arising from the base. Upper surface is shiny, slightly pubescent underneath. Inflorescence in axillary and terminal panicle, flowers are white or creamy-white. The fruit is ovate and blackish-violet in colour.

Benefits:

Excellent for post-partum healing, antiseptic, calming, stimulates appetite, treats colds, rheumatism, kidney disorders.

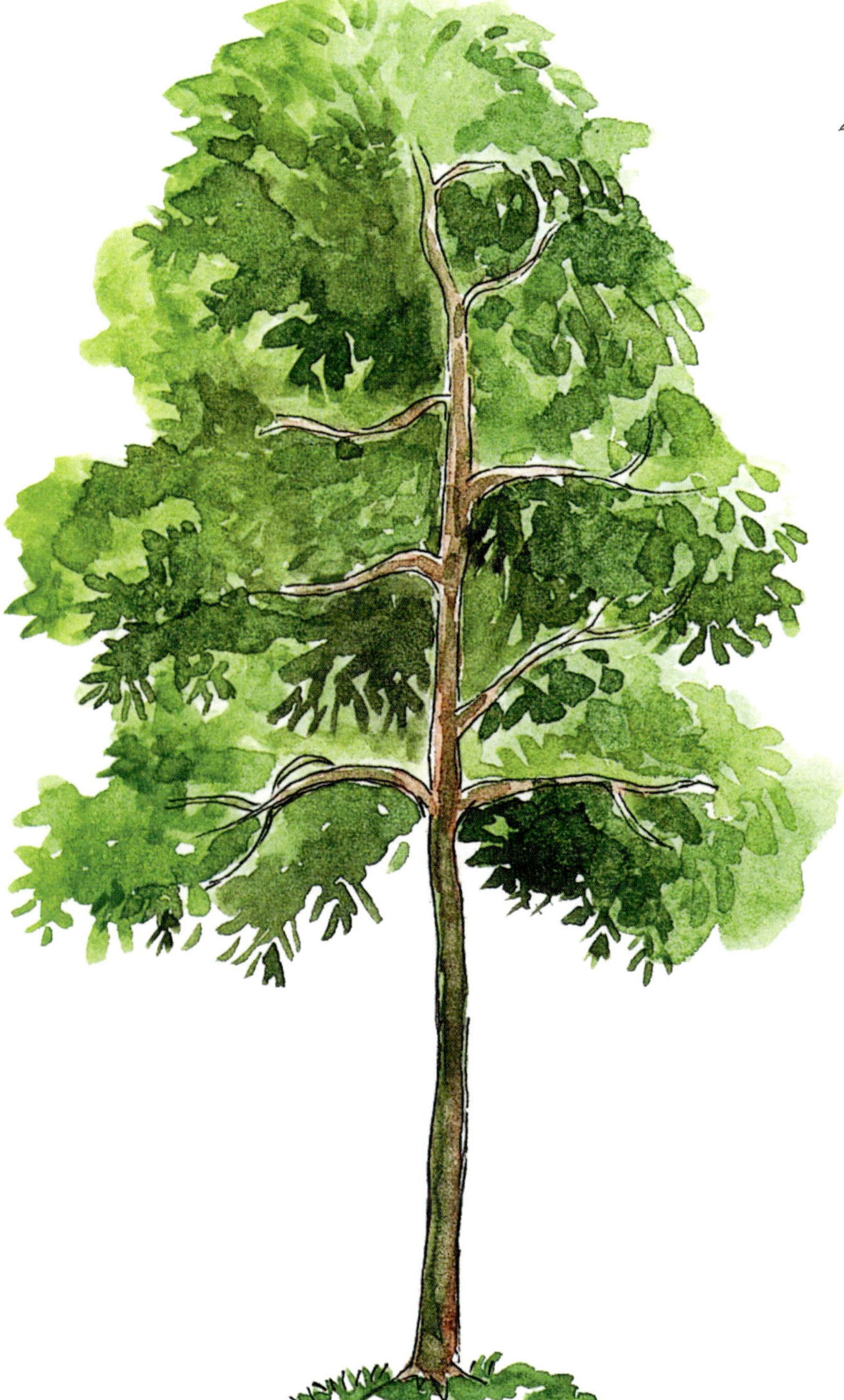

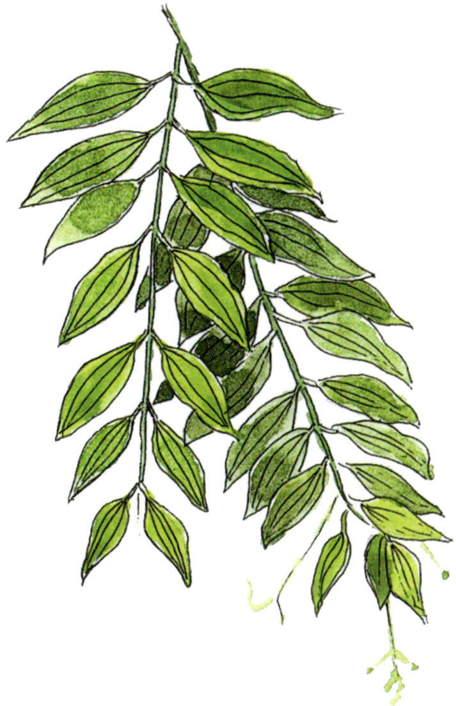

26. *Curcuma longa Linn.*

Family: *Zingiberaceae*

English name: Tumeric

Vernacular name / Local name: *khi-min*

Name in Lao script: ຂີ້ມີ້ນ

Part used in saunas: rhizome & leaves

Description:

Tumeric is a small plant growing in groups separate single stems, approximately 50cm tall. The long, multiple leaves encase the stem, have smooth tapering blades from base to apex and long petioles. The flowers appear on a shoot borne by the centre of the stem. They are whitish-yellow, inserted within an involucre of pale green bracts at base and whitish-pale violet or whitish-yellow bracts at tip. Underneath the ground is the rhizome, distinctly yellow to orange in colour when sliced.

Benefits:

Stimulates circulation, treats arthritis, inflamation, muscular aches and pains, anorexia, sluggish liver, antioxidant, analgesic, improves appetite and digestion, helps to treat scars and skin beauty.

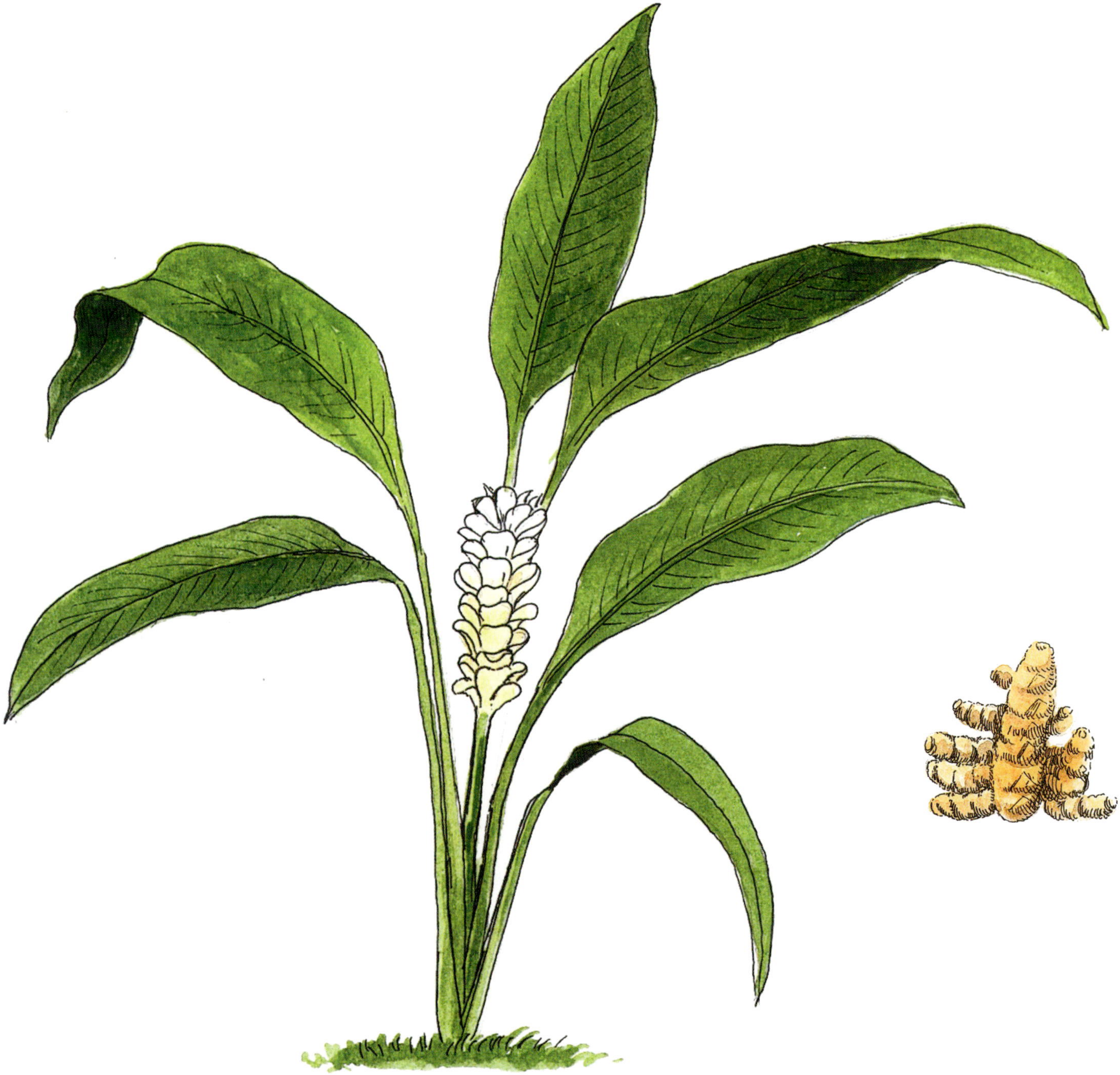

27. *Dalbergia cochinchinensis P.*

Family: *Papilionaceae*

English name: Lao Rosewood

Vernacular/Local name: *pa-dong khaao*

Name in Lao script: ປະດົງຂາວ

Part used in saunas: leaves

Description:

A medium to large evergreen tree 15-30 cm tall. Compound leaves up to 25 cm long with 7-9 leafets, ovate, coriaceous and glabrous, whose reticulate veins are more evident below. The flowers are small and white, 5-6 mm, and are grouped in terminal or axillary panicles. Fruits in the form of a flat pod, 5-6 cms long, with very thin and fragile coat.

Benefits:

Rheumatism.

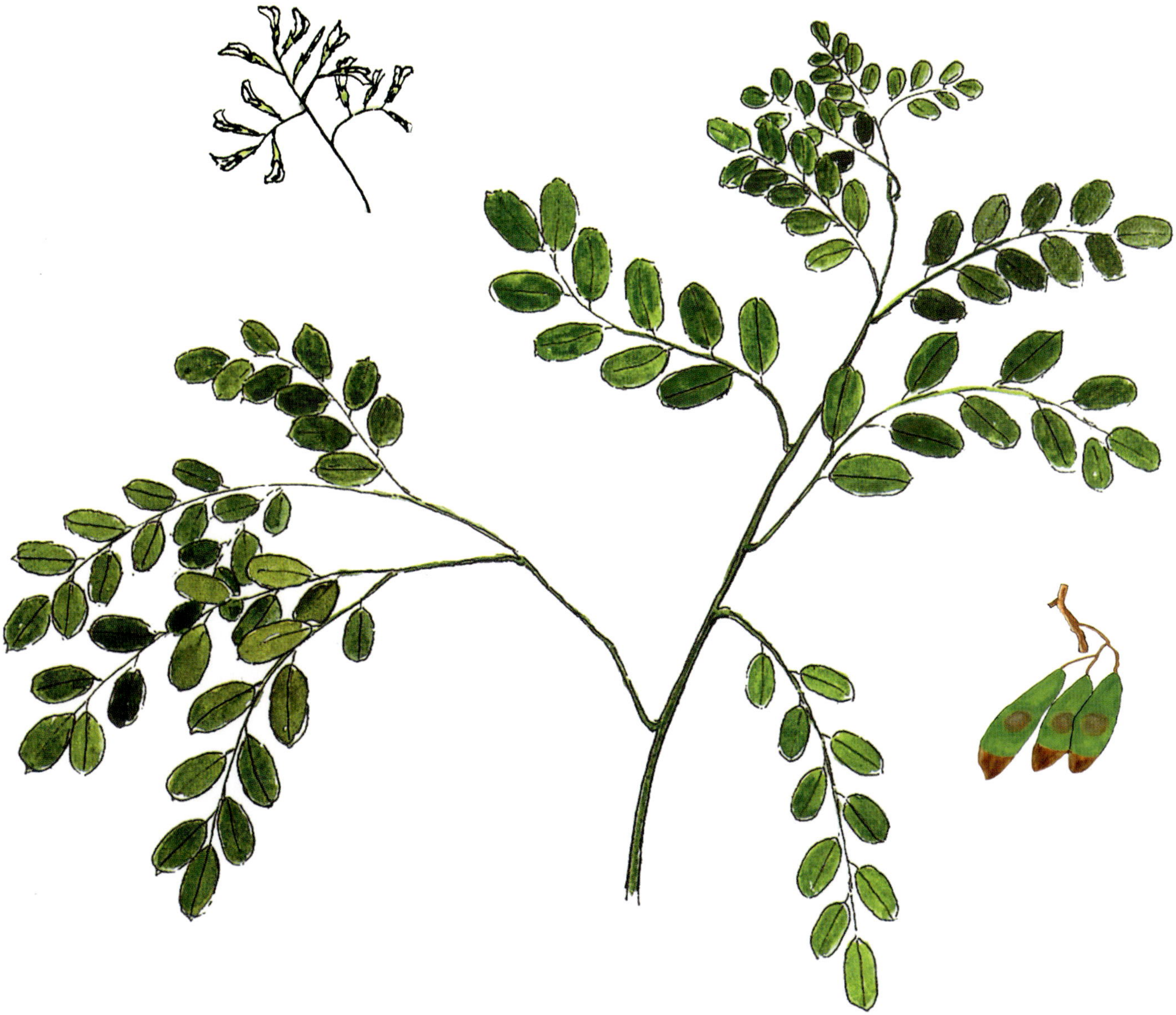

28. *Desmodium trifolium* (L.) DC.

Family: *Papilionaceae*

English name: Tick trefoil, Tick clover (gen.)

Vernacular name / Local name: *pa-dong mot liin*

Name in Lao script: ປະດົງມົດລີ້ນ

Part used in saunas: leaves

Description:

A small perennial herb, 10-30 cm in length, creeping on the ground. The stem is velutinous, pale reddish at the base and light green at the top. Leaves trifoliate or 1-foliate. The terminal leaflet is obovate, obcordate or obovate and rounded, with acute stipule at petiole base. Petiole and blade are velutinous. Flowers are violet or blue-violet and grouped from 2 to 4. Fruits appear as a flat pod, usually curved.

Benefits:

Chickenpox, wounds, boils, skin rashes, abscesses, ulcers, dizziness.

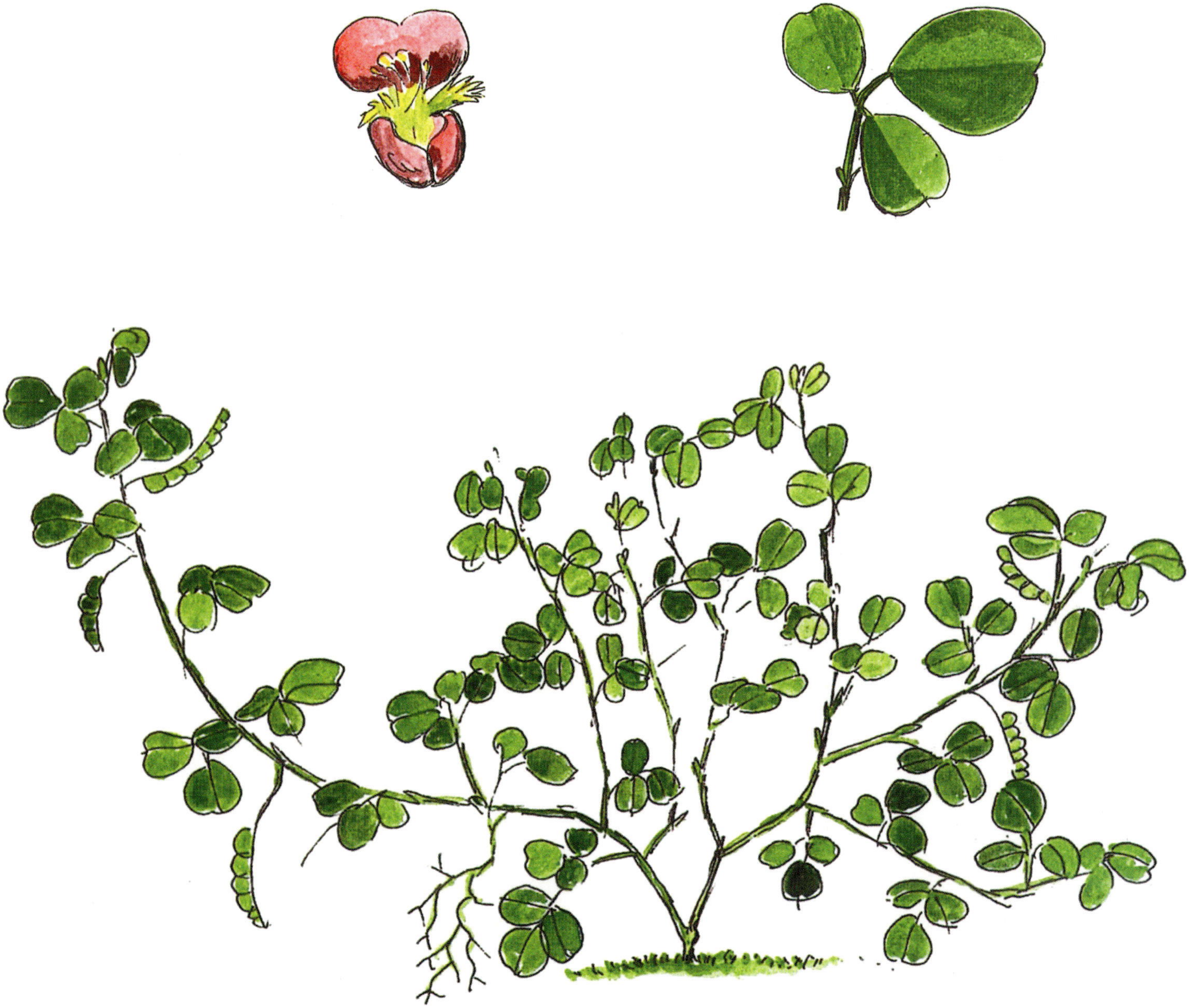

29. *Helixanthera parasitica Lour.*

Family: *Loranthaceae*

English name: ——

Vernacular name / Local name: *phaak mai*

Name in Lao script: ຜາກໄມ້

Part used in saunas: leaves

Description:

A parasitic plant growing on host plants particularly mango trees, jack fruit trees and sugar apple trees. The plant grows to a length of 1-2 m with young twigs being yellow-green and becoming brownish at maturity. The leaves are simple and coriaceous, with oblong or wide lanceolate. They alternate, are glabrous and cuneate at base, acuminate at the tip with a pale green colour. Inflorescence occurs in a dense reddish spike and is axillary. The flowers are rapidly deciduous.

Benefits:

These parasites must occur on a particular tree species to have medicinal properties and as such are rare. For example, when the plants grow on citrus trees, they have medicinal properties that can cure paralysis, stimulate appetite, treat rheumatism, dizziness, spleen disorders.

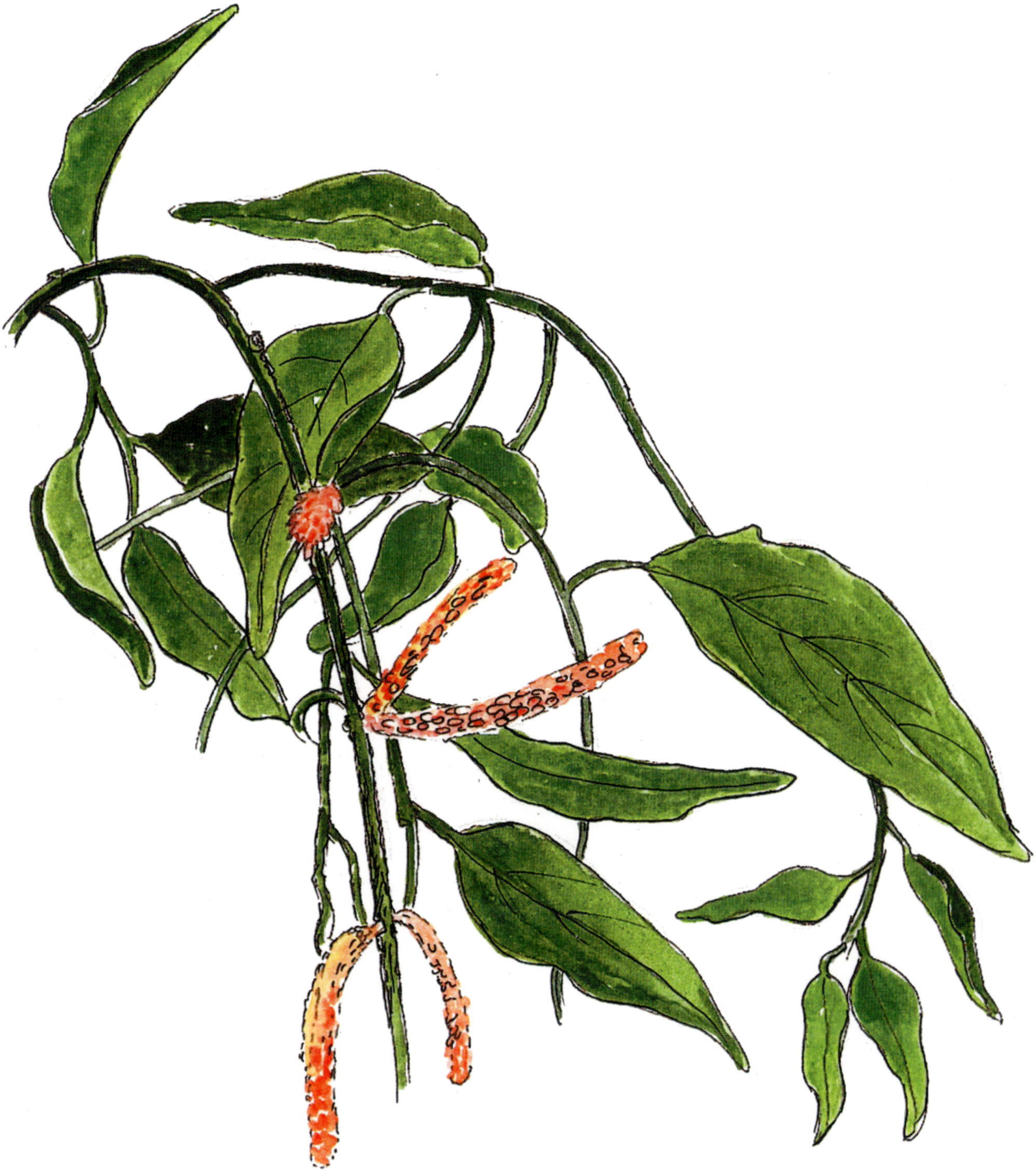

30. *Passiflora foetida L.*

Family: *Passifloraceae*

English name : Stinking passion flower

Vernacular name / Local name: *phak buang*

Name in Lao script: ຜັກບົ້ວງ

Part used in saunas: leaves

Description:

A small climber growing in any free space. Stem slightly hairy, leaves simple and lobed with tendril at the nodes. Flowers are solitary at nodes along the stem. They are white with green bracts and divided in numerous linear lobes. The flowers persist over the fruiting period. Fruit is green becoming orange when ripe.

Benefits:

Calms the nervous system, promotes good sleep, soothes inflammation & itching.

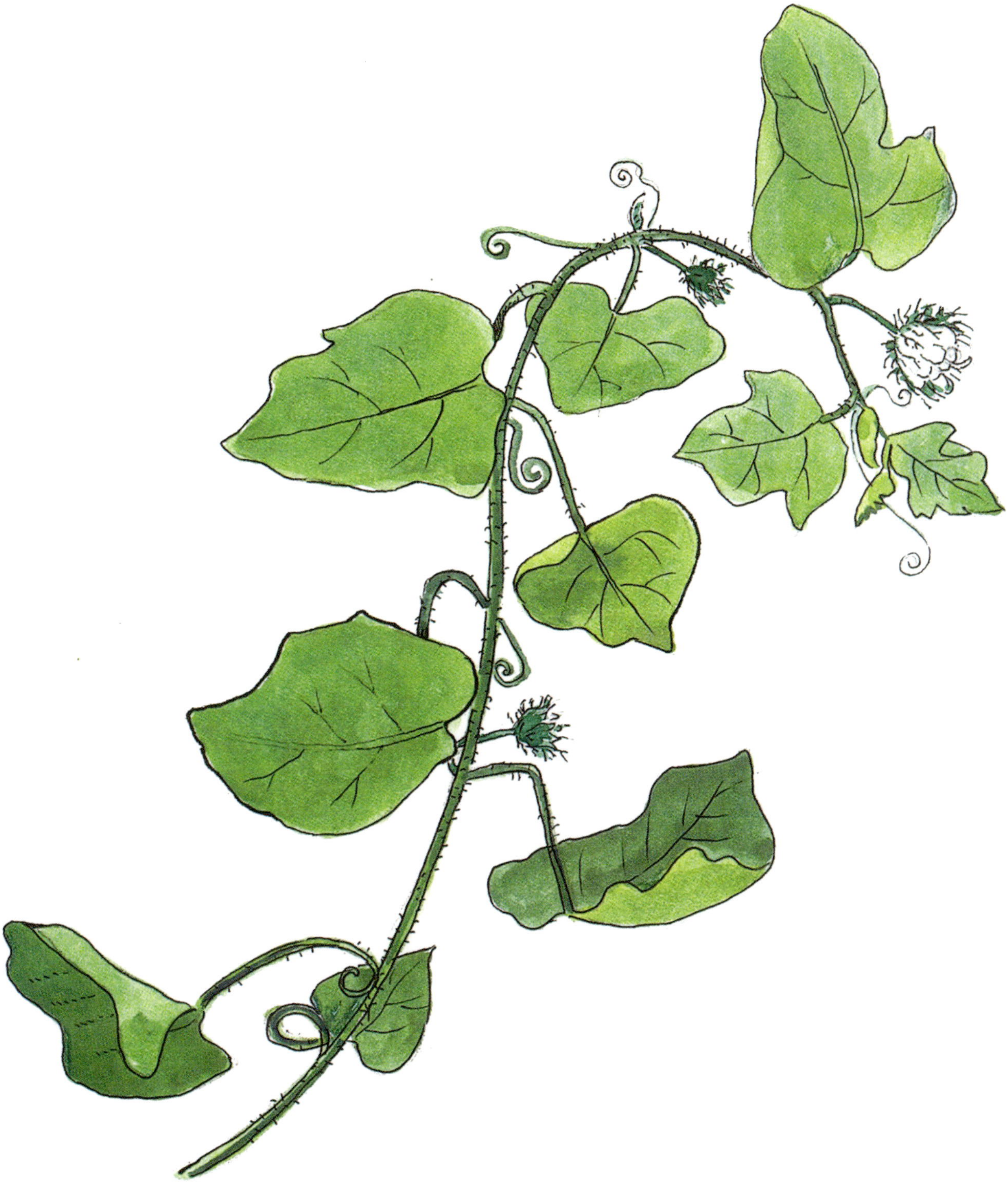

31. *Polygonum odoratum Lour.*

Family: *Polygonaceae*

English name: Vietnamese coriander, Asian mint

Vernacular name / Local name: *phak phaehw*

Name in Lao script: ພັກແຜວ

Part used in saunas: leaves

Description:

A perennial herbaceous plant of 20-30 cm. Stem erect, cylindrical, reddish, glabrous and swollen at the node. Leaves are alternate, lanceolate, glabrous, 1.5-2 cm wide and 4-6 cm long. The petiole is 2-4 mm long, with a red ring at the base and a membranous stipule. Inflorescence is in an axillary and terminal spike with small white flowers. The young leaves are used in cooking as well.

Benefits:

Migraines, fever, nausea, diuretic, indigestion, flatulence & stomach problems.

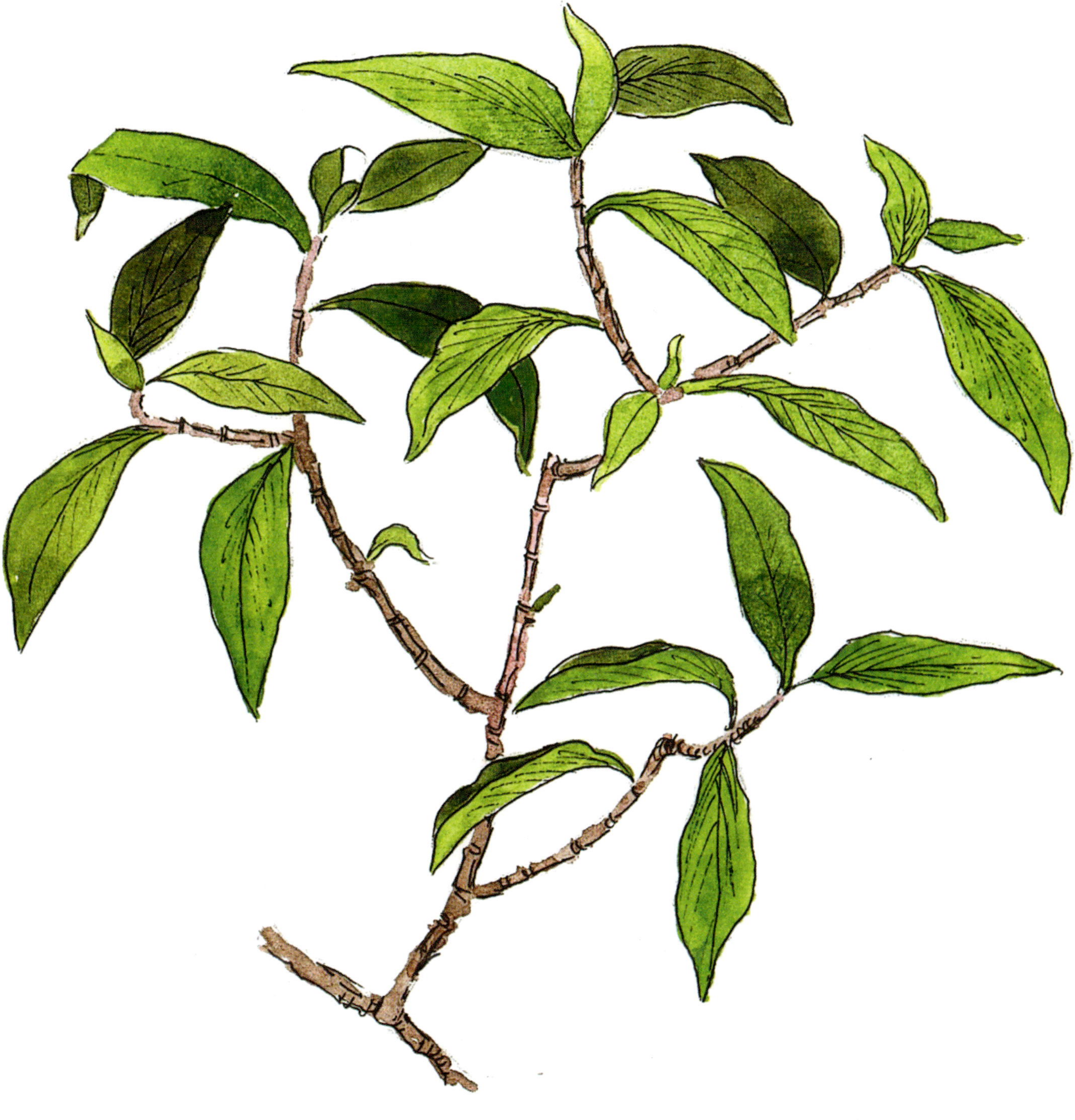

32. *Tinospora crispa (Linn.)Miers ex Hook.f*

Family: *Menispermaceae*

English name: ——

Vernacular name / Local name: *kheua khao hohr*

Name in Lao script: ເຄືອເຂົ້າຮໍ

Part used in saunas: stem and leaves

Description:

A woody climber, usually growing on a tree in dense forest, with a hanging warty-like stem and aerial roots. Leaves are cordate, with thick and shiny dark green blades and long petioles up to 5 cm. Flowers are small and yellowish. Fruits become orange when ripe. The whole plant is very bitter.

Benefits:

Stomach ailments, general tonic, analgesic, blood purifier, disinfectant, gonorrhea, wounds, antimalarial, promotes longevity.

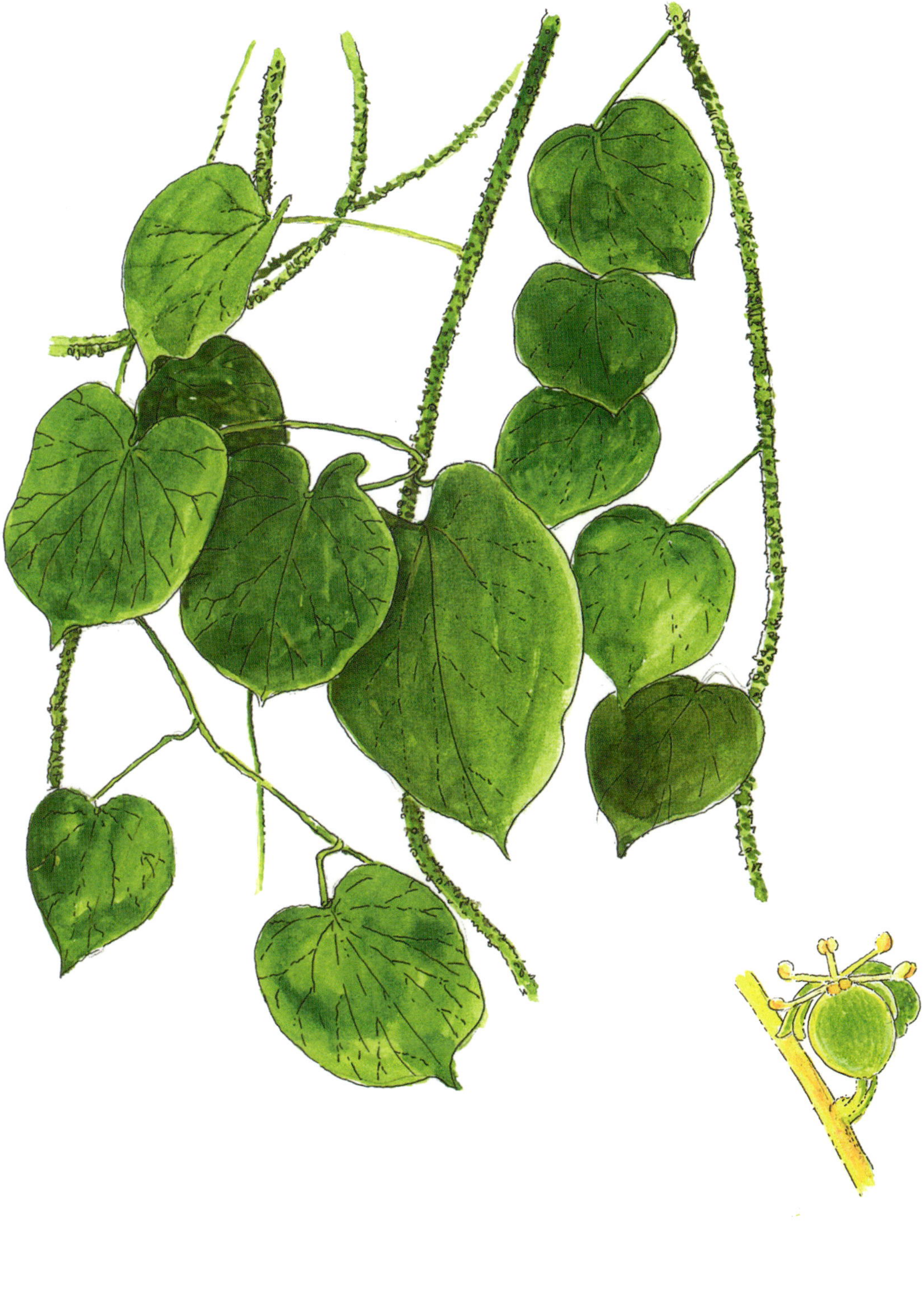

33. Old red ants' nest

Red ants, sometimes called acid ants, are about 1 cm long and live in trees. They build their nests by uniting leaves (but rarely compound leaves because of their size) which they glue together with a net of white secretions produced by the ants. Red ants are well known for their acid secretions that are used for pharmaceutical purposes. The abandoned old nests are used in the sauna.

Benefits:

The old red ants' nest is excellent for relieving dizziness and nausea.

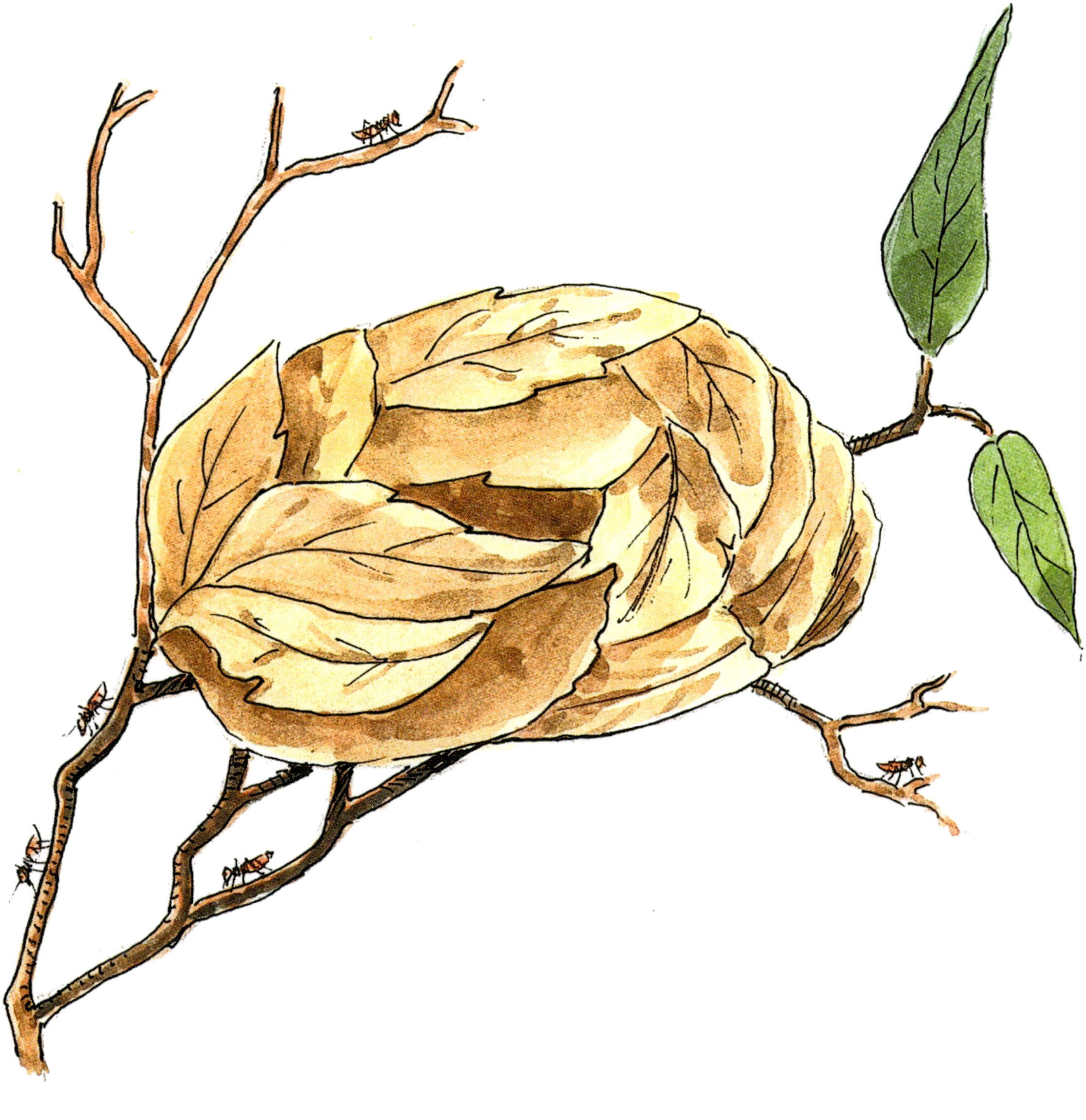

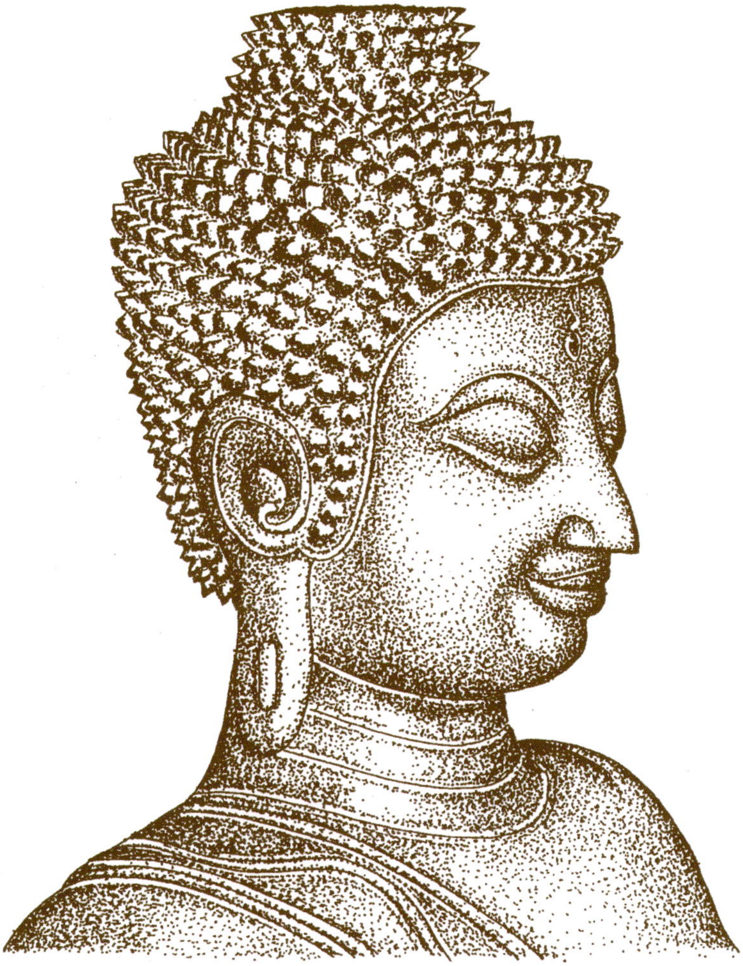

HEALING THE MIND

THE MIND

The mind is a term commonly used to describe the higher functions of the brain, particularly those of which we are subjectively conscious, such as personality traits, emotion, reason, memory, intelligence and thought. Although other species of animals share many of these mental capacities, the term is usually reserved for humans, who seem to have more highly developed faculties than other species.

In the last thirty years, researchers have used modern scientific methods to explore the complex interconnections between mind and body. Their findings suggest that mood, attitude, belief and social status do affect virtually every chronic illness. Emotions such as fear and cynicism, or a sense of hopelessness, can have a detrimental effect on health; whereas courage, good humor, a sense of control, and hopefulness can all be beneficial. It seems that optimistic people are less likely to become ill in the first place and when they do become ill, they tend to live longer and suffer less. Mind/body research has shown, over and over again, that different states of mind directly effect physical wellbeing, mainly through the autonomic nervous system and the glands. The goal of healing is, therefore, not only to bring strength and stability to the physical body but to assist the mind in developing a calm, positive and open perspective.

The science of serenity

This mind/body approach to medicine is already deep rooted in the traditional health systems of South East Asia and it is not uncommon for Lao monasteries to offer psychological, as well as health, services to the community at large. Their "stress busting" techniques could just as easily be found in the latest journals of scientific research since they include relaxation, preventative health practices, physical activity through community service, a sense of spiritual balance via positive thinking, study and meditation; as well as social support and counselling. All these activities contribute significantly to robust health, mental stability and happiness. They come under the modern heading of mind/body medicine, which respects and improves each person's capacity for self-care and self-knowledge.

Meditation

To this end the monastic community regularly offers spiritual teachings and meditation training to the lay community. By sharing their knowledge and offering practical tools for handling the stresses of everyday life, they help people to calm down, to develop insight into their lives and to take a fresh look at the world around them. Alongside their meditation practices, participants are also encouraged to read inspirational literature, to discuss their problems with friends in the community, or one of the monks or nuns, to utilize the health services offered in the temple, to give a little time in selfless service, and to work on developing a happier attitude to life.

Although there are several Buddhist Schools and they focus on various different types of meditation, two methods are common to all and these are Samatha, Tranquillity meditation, and Vipassana, Insight meditation. In Laos these methods of meditation are taught according to the Theravada School of Buddhism, which is the national religion of the country.

Nuns in South East Asia

Nuns in Laos are known as *mae-khaao*. They observe 8-10 precepts and wear white robes with shaved heads. They are not in fact fully ordained nuns, or *bhikkhunis*, since full ordination for women gradually died out in the Theravada tradition.

Full ordination of nuns began during the Buddha's lifetime, when he himself ordained the first women into his monastic order. Traditionally nuns observe 311 precepts and wear similar robes to monks. They also perform the same duties and lead a similar lifestyle.

There is a movement to revive the tradition of fully ordained nuns in the Theravada tradition and there are now *bhikkhunis* from Sri Lanka, Thailand and Burma.

Tranquillity Meditation (Samatha)

Tranquillity meditation is not unique to Buddhism and has been practiced by meditative traditions for centuries. The method involves, first, relaxing the mind into the present moment and then focusing the mind on a single subject or object. The practice of letting go of tensions in the body and mind goes to the very root of healing. There are many techniques for this type of meditation. One of them involves sitting quietly while observing one's breath flow in and out; another focuses on an external object such as a pebble, holy picture or candle. Others suggest concentrating the mind while walking slowly up and down a path, noticing the details of each step and the process of walking. As soon as there is an attempt to limit the mind to one topic in this way, a never-ending stream of thoughts and feelings seem to arise, crowding in to disturb the concentration. These thoughts and feelings have always been there but have not really been observed before. However, with persistence and practice the mind relaxes and clears, settling down into a state of inner peace and tranquillity. Buddhists believe that this is the natural state of the mind.

The condition of the mind is sometimes compared to an ocean, with waves and disturbances on the surface while the depths remain always calm. The idea of this type of meditation is to identify with a deeper, calmer level of mind and just to let the surface condition be as it is, without the least attachment to its being either calm or disturbed.

Vipassana or Insight Meditation

This type of practice was taught by the Buddha and is a profound contribution to the field of meditation. The purpose of Vipassana meditation is to build on the calm and stable state achieved through Samatha, by practicing minute to minute observations of the mind, and the environment, while resting in tranquillity. This system of quietly noticing what is happening as it is happening is called "mindfulness". It consists of peacefully observing the flow of events, thoughts, habits, patterns of behavior and ways we perceive our world, without judgment and without attachment. Through this deep observation, we notice how the mind really works and how we can work with it directly. Penetrative insights spontaneously arise, insights into the way things really are rather than the way we generally perceive them to be. The ultimate goal of Buddhist meditation is to realize a profound state of wisdom where ignorance, and its associated suffering, is permanently eliminated. At the very least this meditation helps us develop a more optimistic and responsible perception of the world, promoting positive emotions, compassionate actions and a sense of appreciation for the interdependence of all life.

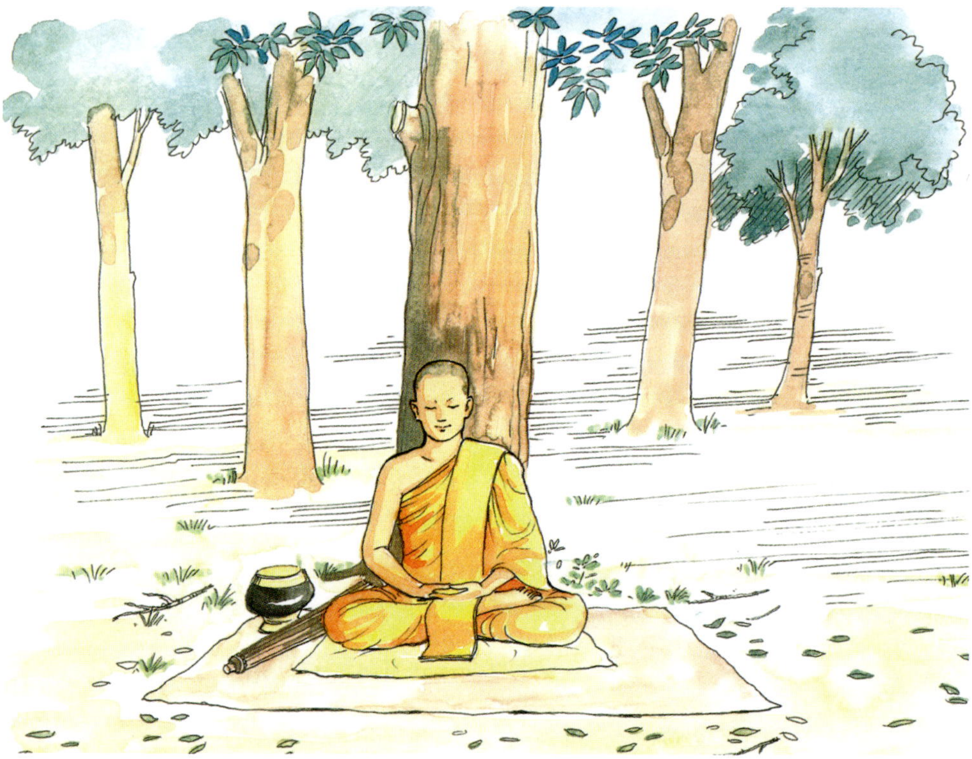

SUMMING UP

The concept that the mind is important in the treatment of illness is integral to the healing approaches of Buddhism, Ayurveda and traditional Chinese medicine, dating back more than 2,000 years. While this integrated approach has been maintained in the traditional healing systems of the East, early scientific developments in the Western world, particularly during the 16th–17th centuries, led to a clear separation between physical and spiritual concerns. Technological advances of that time revealed an observable cellular world, which seemed far removed from the realm of religion, superstition and psychological states. The discovery of bacteria, and then antibiotics, further dispelled the notion that beliefs, or mental states, could influence health. Curing the sick appeared to be a matter for science and technology alone. This effectively separated mind and body, which persisted in Western medicine for centuries to follow.

Over the past 20 years, however, new scientific research into mind-body medicine has emerged and it is providing considerable evidence that psychological factors do, after all, play a substantive role in the development and progression of disease. Many neurologists and psychologists now agree that the mind and body are more intimately connected than was previously thought, and that the well being of one seems directly related to the well being of the other. New and more powerful microscopes have shown that there are minute nerve synapses connecting the body and mind in ways that were not known to exist until recently. By observing the activity of these minute synapses, it is seen that disturbances in the body do affect brain function and, likewise, disturbances in the brain send biochemical shockwaves throughout the body systems.

When using this knowledge in a practical way, it now appears that mind-body interventions, such as focused breathing exercises or meditation, can greatly enhance the effect of standard rehabilitation in many areas. In addition, a combination of stress management and behavioral counselling, as well as relaxation therapy, may be appropriate complementary treatments for coronary disease and some pain-related disorders, like arthritis. Holistic therapies are also effective in the management of various chronic conditions and when offered before surgery, they also seem to improve recovery time and reduce pain following surgical procedures. The physical and emotional risks of using such therapies are minimal and, once tested and standardized, most mind-body interventions can be easily taught.

The results of this type of research are now frequently published in the modern media and are stimulating a lot of public interest. Patients are increasingly interested in integrating both traditional and modern medical treatments into their health care systems. So from the perspective of mind-body interventions the future looks good.

In the area of herbal medicines however, the picture is not as positive and the reason for this is the rapid degradation of natural habitats worldwide. Herbalists and traditional healers have always drawn on nearby forests and fields for the harvesting of their fresh medicinal plants but sadly this is becoming increasingly difficult.

As natural habitats are destroyed, many plant species face the threat of both local and global extinction. As the rate of this extinction is increasing rather than slowing down, there is an urgent need to take care of the areas in which medicinal plants grow, also to document and share knowledge about their usefulness.

SE Asia is home to some of the Earth's most important flora and fauna but every year more of its forests are converted to other land-uses, further degraded, or fragmented. The resulting landscape supports fewer and fewer species of plants and animals.

Even Laos, which has been spared much of the forest loss experienced in neighboring Vietnam, Thailand, and China, is now losing forest cover and quality at an alarming rate. At the middle of the 20th century forest cover in Laos was around 70 % of the surface area, but today it has shrunk to less than 50%. Unfortunately, much of this remaining forest is severely endangered and degenerated.

The pressures caused by economic development and population growth are placing extraordinary pressure on the country's natural resources. Much of this pressure is due to over grazing by livestock, timber extraction, unsustainable slash and burn agricultural practices, uncontrolled forest fires, infrastructure development, like roads and hydro electric schemes, illegal wildlife trade and the commercial collection of medicinal plants and other forest products at unsustainable levels. It is officially recognised by the Government and its development partners that Laos' natural resources are being used up and face serious threats of further depletion in future.

Although such pressures on the environment are high, there are some unique opportunities for Laos to secure a future based on development, but with sound ecological planning. The nation has a relatively low population density and, because of its previous isolation, has had less exposure to pressure from global markets than its neighboring countries. The Lao government's ecological policy involving local people in land-use planning and protected area management could help to prevent future conflicts over resource use.

A program of education to raise public awareness is vital to support these efforts, both in schools and communities all over the country. There is also an urgent need to stimulate widespread interest in conservation before Laos loses the bulk of its natural resources like many of its neighbors.

As a direct result of its rich bio-diversity, Laos still retains resources for traditional healers who can, in spite of everything, find a wide variety of medicinal plants growing in the forests around them.

If we could really understand, and publicize, their usefulness perhaps we might act more urgently to protect the precious forests in which they thrive and find ways to incorporate more plant medicines into our modern medical systems. In this way we would continue to build on the important knowledge of plant medicines that we already have.

I hope this book will encourage people to actively support the protection of their natural resources and to insist on a more integrated approach to health care from their doctors. Changes in attitude, particularly in the area of medicine, are slow and frequently demand driven. The more patients expect an integrated approach to their health care, the more they will get it. The forests of Laos and the world could benefit greatly from this.

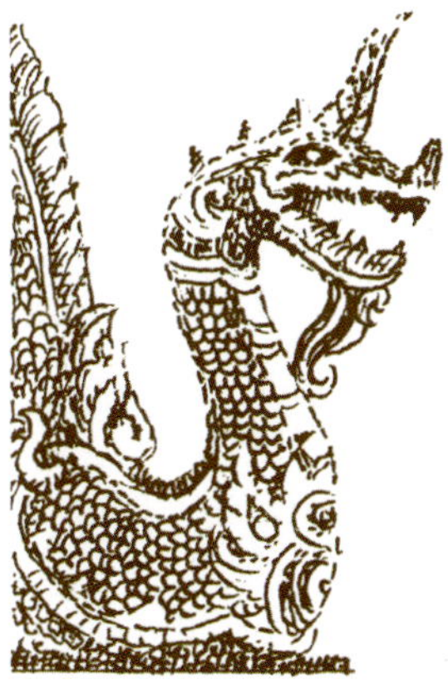

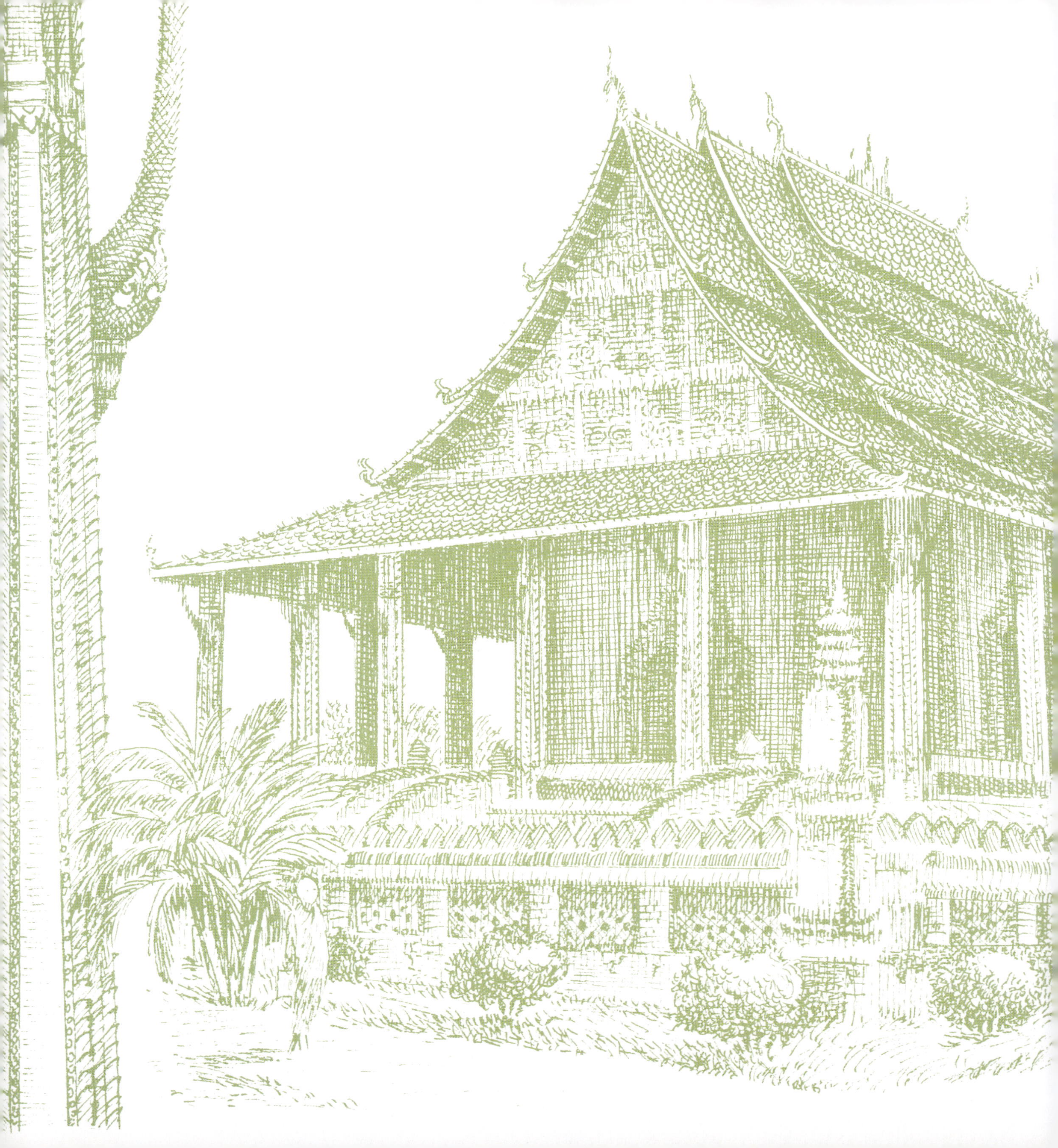

APPENDIX

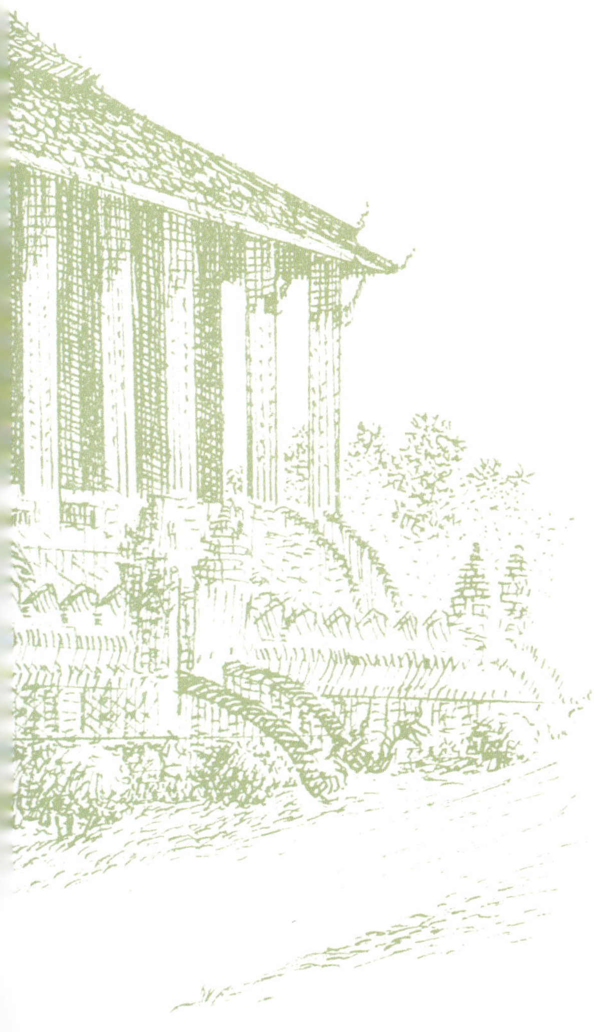

PLANTS USED DAILY

No	Lao Script	Lao phonetics	Common Name	Family	Scientific
1	ອີ່ຕູ່ນາ, ຈີ່ນາຍກ້ອມ	I-tuu naa or Ji-naai kohrm		Scrophulariaceae	Adenosma bracteosum Bon.
2	ຕົ້ນໝາດໃຫຍ່, ຕົ້ນໝາດຫຼວງ	Ton naat nyai or ton naat luang	Camphor tree	Asteraceae	Blumea balsamifera DC
3	ຕົ້ນຂີ່ຫູດ	Ton khi-huut	Leech Lime	Rutaceae	Citrus hystrix DC.
4	ຕົ້ນໝາກກ້ຽງ	Ton mak-kiang	Sweet Orange	Rutaceae	Citrus sinensis (L.) Osb.
5	ຕົ້ນເປົ້າໃຫຍ່, ຕົ້ນເປົ້າ	Ton pao nyai or ton pao		Euphorbiaceae	Croton roxburghii Balakor.
6	ສີໄຄເຄື່ອງ	Sii khai kheuang	Citronella	Poaceae	Cymbopogon nardus Rendle
7	ຕົ້ນວິກ	Ton vik	Blue Gum or Eucalyptus	Myrtaceae	Eucalyptus globulus Labill.

	Part used	Frequency	Benefits
	Whole plant with flowers	Daily	Respiratory ailments, herbal bathing after childbirth, analgesic, anti-inflammatory, skin beauty.
	Leaves	Always include daily	Heartburn & indigestion, treats insomnia, hypertension, antispasmodic, stimulates sweating, respiratory ailments & asthma, antibacterial, stomach problems, headaches, dizziness, joint pains.
	Leaves	Daily	Stimulant, stomach ache, blood purifier, good for hair & skin, respiratory congestion.
	Leaves	Daily	Coughs, colds, expectorant, anorexia, stomacic, dizziness and nausea, cooling and calming
	Leaves	Daily	Anti-toxic, cleanses the blood, prevents blood clots, bactericidal, treats nausea, helps body retain minerals, diarrhea, flatulence, vomiting.
	Leaves & bulb	Daily	Post heart attack, calming, menstrual problems, flatulance, vomiting, rheumatism, fevers, kills intestinal parasites, antiseptic, insect repellent.
	Leaves	Daily	Strong antibacterial action, wounds and skin problems, respiratory ailments and fevers, opens pores & promotes sweating.

No	Lao Script	Lao phonetics	Common Name	Family	Scientific
8	ຕົ້ນຊົມຊື່ນ	Ton som seuhn	Jamaica mandarin orange	Rutaceae	Glycosmis pentaphylla Correa.
9	ເຄືອເອັນອ່ອນ	Kheua en ohrn	Black creeper	Apocynaceae	Ichnocarpus Frutescens (L.) W.T. Aiton
10	ພັກຂະແຍງ	Phak kha-nyaehng	Bug herb	Scrophulariaceae	Limnophila geoffrayi Bon.
11	ສາລະນາດ, ກາລະບຸນ	Saalanat, kaalabuun	Japanese mint	Lamiaceae	Mentha arvensis Linn.
12	ໃບພັກອີ່ຕູ່ແລ້ ກະເພົາແດງ	Phak i-tuu laeh, ka-phao daehng	Holy or sacred Basil	Lamiaceae	Ocimum sanctum L. (red variety)
13	ຫຍ້າມຸ້ງກະຕ່າຍ	Nyaa mung ka-taai		Rubiaceae	Oldenlandia capitellata O.Kze
14	ຕົ້ນໝາກຂາມສົ້ມ	Ton mak-khaam som	Tamarind	Ceasalpiniaceae	Tamarindus indica Linn.
15	ພີເສືອນ້ອຍ	Phi-seua noi	Indian wild pepper	Verbenaceae	Vitex trifolia L.

	Part used	Frequency	Benefits
	Leaves	Always include daily	Synergistic relationship with Camphor (*ton naat*), controls itchiness, assists in post-partum depression, anorexia, headaches, skin beauty.
	Leaves & vine stems	Daily	Strengthens and maintains the nervous system, relieves paralysis, tonic.
	Whole plant and flowers	Daily	Dizziness, calming, flatulance, antispasmodic.
	leaves	Daily	Calms nervous system, respiratory ailments, anti-toxic, induces sweating, gastric upsets, headache.
	Leaves	Daily	Lacto-stimulant, respiratory ailments, nerve tonic, muscular pain, laxative.
	Leaves	Daily	Nausea, vomiting, dizziness, flatulence.
	Leaves	Daily	Rheumatism, cough and phlegm, sores and wounds, conjunctivitis, constipation, calming. Skin beauty: fruit pulp on skin during sauna.
	Leaves	Daily	Reduces swelling eg - after childbirth, rheumatism, wounds, fever, cough & mucus, diuretic.

PLANTS USED OCCASIONALLY

No	Lao Script	Lao phonetics	Common name	Family name	Scientific name
16	ຕົ້ນໝາກນາວ	Ton mak-naao	Common Lime, Key Lime or Mexican Lime	Rutaceae	Citrus aurantifolia Swing.
17	ຫູເສືອ	Huu seua	Indian borage	Lamiaceae	Coleus ambonicus Lour.
18	ໜາດເໝົ່າ	Naat nao		Asteraceae	Conyza aurita L.f.
19	ຕົ້ນສະມັດ	Ton sa-mat	Lime berry, orange berry, butterfly tree	Rutaceae	Micromelum hirsutum Oliv.
20	ພັກອີ່ຕູ່ໃຫຍ່	Phak i-tuu nyai	Hairy Basil	Lamiaceae	Ocimum gratissimum Linn.
21	ພັກອີ່ຕູ່ຂຽວນ້ອຍ, ກະເພົາຂາວ	Phak i-tuu khiao noi, ka-phao khaao	White holy basil or sacred basil	Lamiaceae	Ocimum sanctum L. (white variety)
22	ຫວານໄພ	Vaan phai	Chinese ginger	Zingiberaceae	Zingiber purureum Rosc.

	Part used	Frequency	Benefits
	Leaves	Occasionally	Sedative, fever, nausea, dizziness, expectorant, asthma, improves circulation, colds, acne, infections, detoxification, anti-inflammatory. Improves menstruation, stimulates sweating.
	Leaves	Occasionally	Overheating especially in children, treats wounds, headaches, coughs, stomach ailments.
	Leaves	Occasionally	Excellent for post-partum healing.
	Leaves	Occasionally	Treats boils, tightens sagging flesh, assists in post-partum healing.
	Leaves	Occasionally	Antispasmodic, antidepressant, nerve tonic, warming, restorative, treats stomach ailments.
	Leaves	Occasionally	Sedative and antidepressant, nerve tonic, fever, lacto-stimulant, muscular and diuretic, induces menstruation, laxative.
	Stems, leaves and rhizome	Occasionally	Fainting, indigestion.

PLANTS USED FOR SPECIAL AILMENTS

No	Lao Script	Lao phonetics	Common name	Family name	Scientific name
23	ຕົ້ນຕີນເປັດ	Ton tiin pet	Devil tree	Apocynaceae	Alstonia scholaris R. Br.
24	ຕົ້ນໝາກເຟືອງ	Ton mak-feuang	Star fruit	Oxalidaceae	Averrhoea carambola Linn.
25	ຕົ້ນຈວງ	Ton juang or saa juang	Chinese cassia	Lauraceae	Cinnamomum cassia Bl.
26	ຂີ່ມິນ	Khi-min	Tumeric	Zingiberaceae	Curcuma longa Linn.
27	ປະດົງຂາວ	Pa-dong khaao	Lao rosewood	Papilionaceae	Dalbergia cochinchinensis P.
28	ປະດົງມົດລີ້ນ	Pa-dong mot liin	Tick trefoil, tick clover (gen.)	Papilionaceae	Desmodium trifolium (L.) DC
29	ຜາກໄມ້	Phaak mai		Loranthaceae	Helixanthera parasitica Lour.
30	ພັກບ້ວງ	Phak buang	Stinking passion flower	Passifloraceae	Passiflora foetida L.
31	ພັກແຜວ	Phak phaehw	Vietnamese coriander, Asian mint	Polygonaceae	Polygonum odoratum Lour.
32	ເຄື່ອເຂົ້າຮໍ	Kheua khao hohr		Menispermaceae	Tinospora crispa (Linn.) Miers

	Part used	Frequency	Benefits
	Leaves & bark	Special ailments	Prevents bone loss, indigestion, flatulence, stomach ailments, general tonic, treats malaria, fever, skin diseases, bactericidal.
	Leaves	Special ailments	Chickenpox, ringworm, headache, fever, chills, intestinal disorders.
	Leaves	Special ailments	Excellent for post-partum healing, antiseptic, calming, stimulates appetite, treats colds, rheumatism, kidney disorders,
	Leaves & rhizome	Special ailments	Stimulates circulation, treats arthritis, inflamation, muscular aches and pains, anorexia, sluggish liver, anti-oxidant, analgesic, improves appetite and digestion, skin beauty.
	Leaves	Special ailments	Rheumatism.
	Leaves	Special ailments	Chickenpox, wounds, boils, abscesses, ulcers, dizziness.
	Leaves	Special ailments	Stimulates appetite, treats rheumatism, paralysis, dizziness, spleen disorders.
	Leaves	Special ailments	Treats nervous system, soothes inflammation & itching.
	Leaves	Special ailments	Migraines, fever, nausea, diuretic.
	Leaves & stem	Special ailments	Stomach ailments, general tonic, analgesic, blood purifier, disinfectant, gonorrhea, wounds, antimalarial, promotes longevity.

PLANT TERMINOLOGY

Acuminate	:	tapering to a sharp point and forming concave side along the tip
Acute	:	tapering to a pointed apex
Alternate	:	when a leaf is singly at each node
Apiculate	:	quadrally tapering to a sharp point with concave sides
Axillary	:	when an inflorescence appears between a stem and a leaf petiole or between a stem and another branch.
Biserrate	:	doubly serrate
Cordate	:	heart-shaped
Corolla	:	name of all of the petals of a flower
Crenate	:	with rounded teeth along the margin
Cuneate	:	wedge-shaped triangular and tapering at the base
Deciduous	:	not persistent
Decussate	:	with each pair of leaves at right angles to the other pair.
Dentate	:	toothed along the margin directed outwards
Entire	:	continuous margin of a leaf
1-foliate	:	when one leaflet is present
Follicle	:	dry dehiscent fruit
Glabrous	:	hairless or smooth
Hirsute	:	pubescent with coarse, stiff hairs
Imparipennate	:	pinnately compound with one terminal leaflet
Involucre	:	all of the flowers bracts grouped together at the base of a flower or an inflorescence
Lanceolate	:	lance-shaped
Leaflet	:	a division of a compound leaf
Obcordate	:	inversely cordate
Oblanceolate	:	inversely lanceolate
Oblique	:	unequal blade side
Oblong	:	two to four times longer than broad with nearly parallel sides
Obovate	:	inversely ovate
Opposite	:	when two leaves are across from one another at the same node
Panicle	:	a branched inflorescence with flower maturing from the bottom upwards

Perennial	:	when the plant life is long
Petiole	:	a leaf stalk
Pinnate	:	compound leaf with leaflets arranged on opposite sides of an elongated axis
Pubescent	:	covered with short, soft hairs
Punctate	:	dotted with glands
Raceme	:	an elongated inflorescence with pedicellate flowers maturing from the bottom upwards
Serrate	:	toothed along the margin with the sharp teeth pointing forward
Sessile	:	attached directly without a supporting stalk
Simple	:	when a leaf blade is not separated into leaflets
Sinuate	:	wavy form
Stipule	:	one of pair of leaflet-like appendages found at the base of the petiole of some leaves
Tendril	:	twining organ used to grasp support for climbing
Terminal	:	at the end of the branch
Tomentose	:	with a covering of short or wooly hairs
Trifoliate	:	when a leaf blade is separated in three small leaves or three leaflets
Umbel	:	inflorescence with the pedicels arising more or less from a common point, bearing condensed set of flowers.
Velutinous	:	covered with short, soft, spreading hairs
Verticillated	:	arranged of similar parts around a central axis or whorled

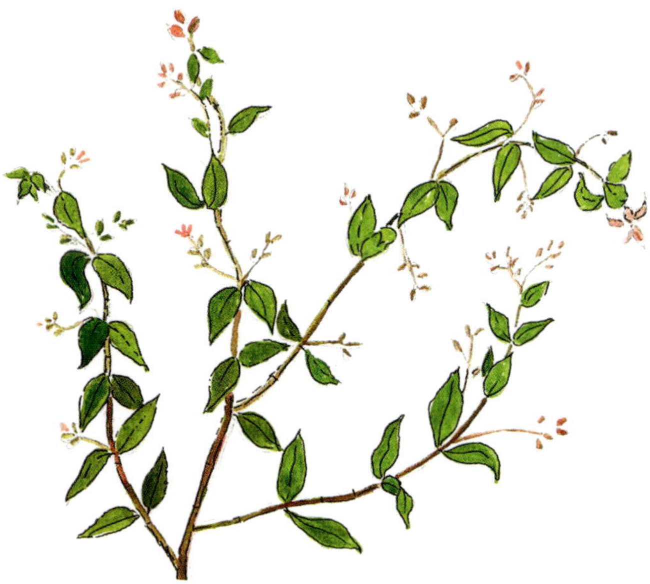

PLANTS LISTED BY FAMILY ORDER

	Daily	Occasionally	Sp. Ailment	Tea	Part used	Page
Acanthaceae						
Andrographis paniculata (Burm.f.) Nees				+		
Apocynaceae						
Alstonia scholaris (L.) R.			+		Leaves & bark	76
Ichnocarpus frutescens (L.) W.T. Aiton	+				Leaves & stem	48
Asteraceae						
Blumea balsamifera (L.) DC.	+				Leaves	34
Conyza aurita L.f.		+			Leaves	66
Caesalpiniaceae						
Tamarindus indica Linn.	+				Leaves & fruits	58
Euphorbiaceae						
Croton roxburghii Balakor.	+				Leaves	40
Lamiaceae						
Coleus ambonicus Lour.		+			Leaves	64
Mentha arvensis Linn.	+				Leaves	52
Ocimum gratissimum Linn.		+			Leaves	70
Ocimum sanctum L. (Red variety)	+				Leaves	54
Ocimum sanctum L. (white variety)		+			Leaves	72
Orthosiphon aristatus Miq.				+	Leaves	
Lauraceae						
Cinnamomum cassia (Nees) Nees & Eberh.			+		Leaves	80
Loranthaceae						
Helixanthera parasitica Lour.			+		Leaves	88
Menispermaceae						
Tinospora crispa (Linn.) Miers ex Hook.f.			+	+	Leaves & stem	94
Myrtaceae						
Eucalyptus globulus Labill.	+				Leaves	44

	Daily	Occasionally	Sp. Ailment	Tea	Part used	Page
Oxalidaceae						
Averrhoa carambola Linn.			+		Leaves	78
Papilionaceae						
Dalbergia Cochinchinensis			+		Leaves	84
Desmodium trifolium (L.) DC.			+		Leaves	86
Passifloraceae						
Passiflora foetida L.			+		Leaves	90
Poaceae						
Cymbopogon citratus (DC.) Stapf				+	Leaves & bulb	42
Cymbopogon nardus Rendle	+				Leaves & bulb	42
Bambusa spp.				+	Leaves	
Polygonaceae						
Polygonum odoratum Lour.			+		Leaves	92
Rubiaceae						
Oldenlandia capitellata O.Kze	+				Leaves	56
Rutaceae						
Citrus aurantifolia (Christm. & Pang) Swing.		+			Leaves	62
Citrus hystrix DC.	+				Leaves	36
Citrus sinensis (L.) Osb.	+				Leaves	38
Glycosmis pentaphylla Corr.	+				Leaves	46
Micromelum minutum(Forst.f.)Wight & Arn.		+			Leaves	68
Scrophulariaceae						
Adenosma bracteosum Bon.	+				Whole plant	32
Limnophila geoffrayi Bon.	+				Whole plant	50
Verbenaceae						
Vitex trifolia L.	+				Leaves	60
Zingiberaceae						
Curcuma longa Linn.			+	+	Leaves, rhizome	82
Zingiber purureum Rosc.		+			Leaves, rhizome	74
Zingiber officinale Rosc.				+	Rhizome	

PLANT INDEX BY SCIENTIFIC NAME

Scientific name	Family name	Local name	Pages
Ocimum sanctum L. (white variety)	Lamiaceae	Phak i-tuu khiao noi or ka-phao khaao	72
Oldenlandia capitellata O.Kze	Rubiaceae	Nyaa mung ka-taai	56
Passiflora foetida L.	Passifloraceae	Phak buang	90
Polygonum odoratum Lour.	Polygonaceae	Phak phaehw	92
Tamarindus indica Linn.	Ceasalpiniaceae	Ton mak-khaam som	58
Tinospora crispa (Linn.) Miers	Menispermaceae	Kheua khao hohr	32
Vitex trifolia L.	Verbenaceae	Phi-seua noi	60
Zingiber purureum Rosc.	Zingiberaceae	Vaan phai	74

BIBLIOGRAPHY

Brown, MacAlister and Joseph J. Zasloff, *Apprentice Revolutionaries: The Communist Movement in Laos, 1930 -1986*; Stanford: Hoover Institute Press, 1986.

Conze, Edward, *Buddhism: Its Essence and Development*; Cambridge: Windhorse Publications, 2004.

Conze, Edward, *Buddhist Thought in India: Three Phases of Buddhist Philosophy*; Ann Arbor: University of Michigan Press, 1967.

Hall, D.G.E., *A History of South East Asia*; London: The Macmillan Press, 1993.

Halpern, Joel M., *Government, Politics, and Social Structure of Laos: A Study in Tradition and Innovation*; Christiansburg, Virginia: Dalley Book Service, 1990.

Herman, A. L., *An Introduction to Buddhist Thought: A Philosophic History of Indian Buddhism*; Lanham: University Press of America, 1984.

Humphreys, Christmas, *Buddhism*; London: Penguin, 1962.

Jumsai, M. L., *The History of Laos* (2nd ed.); Bangkok: Chalermnit, 1971.

Lawless, Julia., *Aromatherapy and the Mind*; London & California: Thorsons Publishers, 1994.

———, *The Illustrated Encyclopedia of Essential Oils: The Complete Guide to the Use of Oils in Aromatherapy and Herbalism*; Rockport: Element Books, 1995.

Le Gadec, Y. La Pharmacopée Laotienne, in *Moniteur d'Indochine*, 599 (1-1930); Hanoi, 1930.

Lopetcharat, Somkiat., *Lao Buddha and its History*; Bangkok: Amarin Printing and Publishing Co., 2000.

Manandhar, Narayan P., *Plants and People of Nepal*; Portland: Timber Press, 2002.

Raju, P. T., *The Philosophical Traditions of India*; London: George Allen & Unwin Ltd., 1971

———, *Structural Depths of Indian Thought*; Albany: SUNY Press, 1985.

Saralamp, Promjit, Terry Clayton, et al, *Medicinal Plants in Thailand* (2 Vols); Bangkok: Faculty of Pharmacy, Mahidol University, 1996/97.

Souvannavong, O., Quelques Pratique de Médicine Traditionnelle, in *France-Asie 118-120*, pp. 975-978; Saigon, 1956.

Tanaka, Dr. Yoshitaka & Dr.Nguyen Van Ke, *Edible Wild Plants of Vietnam: The Bountiful Garden*; Bangkok: Orchid Press, 2007.

[Tibetan Translation Series], *Dhammapada*; Berkeley: Dharma Press, 1985.

Tisserand, Robert B., *The Art of Aromatherapy: The Healing and Beautifying Properties of the Essential Oils of Flowers and Herbs*; Rochester: Healing Arts Press, 1979.

Tiyavanich, Kamala., *Forest Recollections*; Chiang Mai: Silkworm Books, 1997.

———, *The Buddha in the Jungle*; Chiang Mai & Seattle: Silkworm Books & University of Washington Press, 2003.

Valnet, Dr Jean., *The Practice of Aromatherapy*; Saffron Walden: C.W. Daniel Co., 1980.

various, *Journal of Essential Oil Research*, Wheaton: Allured Publishing Corp., 1989-.

Vidal, J.; La Théraputique par les Plantes au Laos, in *Journal d'Agriculture Tropicale et de Botanique Appliquées*, Vol. 10; Paris, 1958.

Viravong, Maha-Sila, *The History of Laos*; New York: Paragon Book Co., 1964.

Watanabe, Takahashi et al, *A Hand Book of Medicinal Plants of Nepal*; Bangkok: Kobfa Publishing, 2005

Worwood, Valarie Ann, *The Fragrant Pharmacy*; London: Bantam Books / Macmillan, 1991.

———, *The Fragrant Mind*; London: Doubleday 1995.

Zysk, Kenneth G., *Asceticism and Healing in Ancient India*; Oxford: Oxford University Press, 1991.

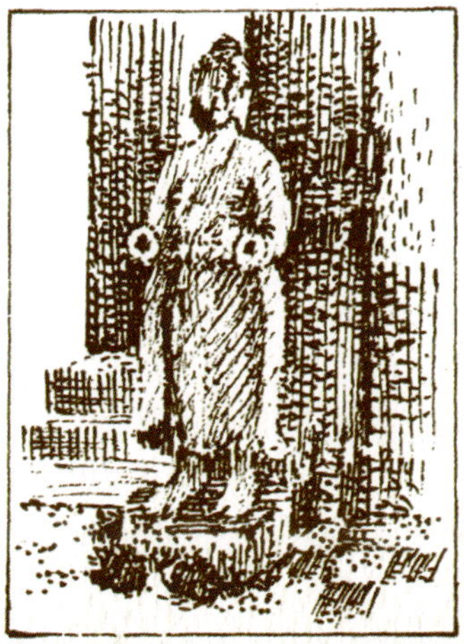

ABOUT THE AUTHOR

DENISE TOMECKO was born and raised in East and Central Africa. Her passion for the untouched beauty of the African wilderness, and her respect for the interconnection of all living things, began with frequent camping trips into the "bush" with her parents. It was during these adventures that she witnessed the seasons and rhythms of nature, spent nights under the stars, and saw how the local tribes lived in harmony with the flora and fauna of their surroundings.

Her interest in healing goes back to childhood when she would mix plant potions to treat imaginary patients. She has since trained as an Aromatherapist, massage therapist, counsellor and has taken courses in other healing methods. She has incorporated her interest in Yoga, Vedantic philosophy and Buddhism into her enthusiasm for the healing arts and preservation of the natural world.

As a Buddhist, Denise studied for many years with prominent Tibetan Lamas and also with other leading Buddhist teachers, both male and female, in the Theravada traditions of Laos and Thailand; the most notable of these being Achann Saly of the Lao Forest Tradition, with whom she studied for four years. These encounters brought a new perspective to her life, opening her mind to the urgent necessity of combining modern material and scientific progress with universal spiritual values and using this as a practical working base in the continuing development of our world.

After meeting her husband Jim in Tanzania, East Africa, Denise has travelled with him for more that 30 years in Africa, Nepal and Laos. She and her husband are now living in Bangkok, Thailand.

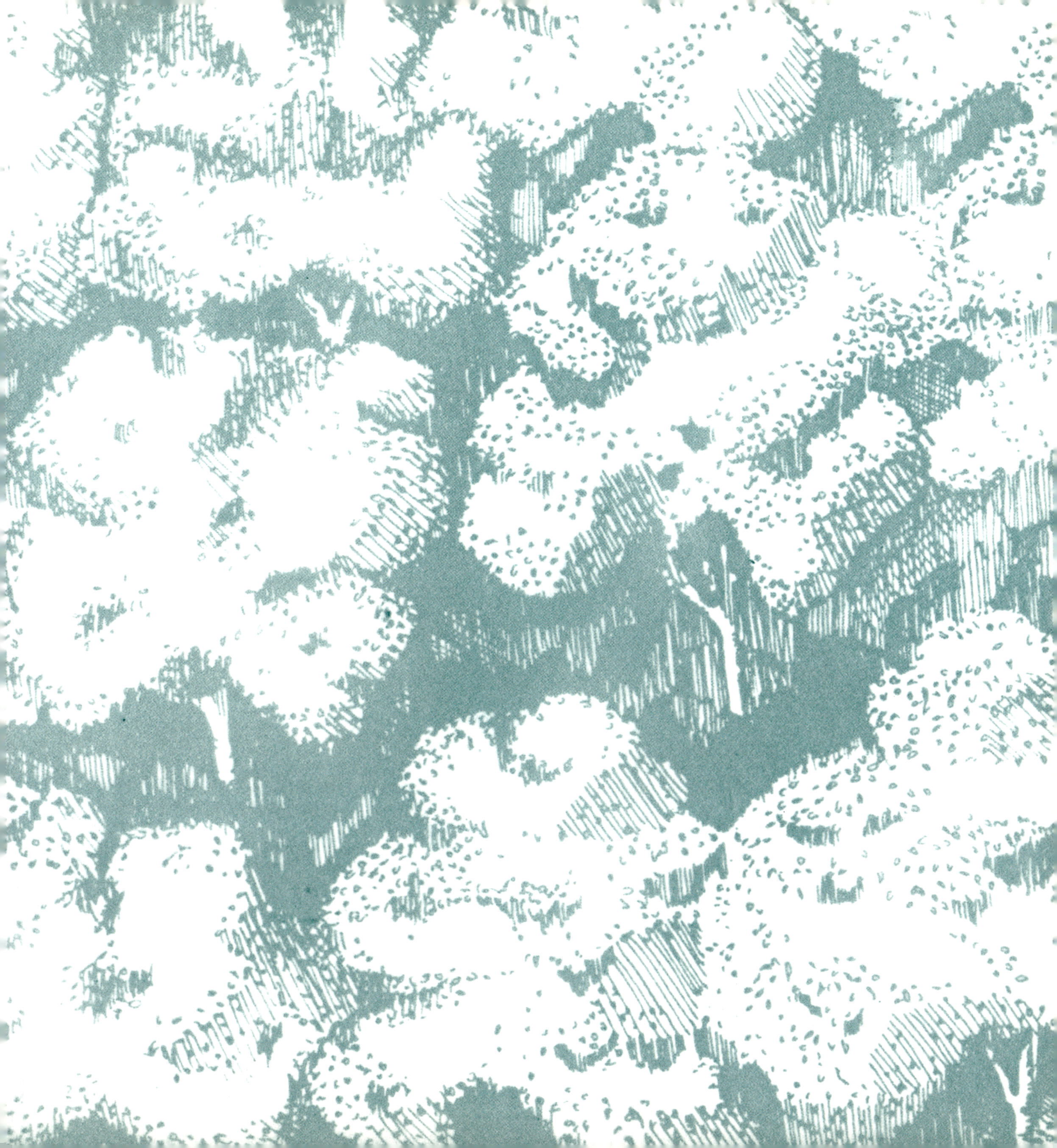

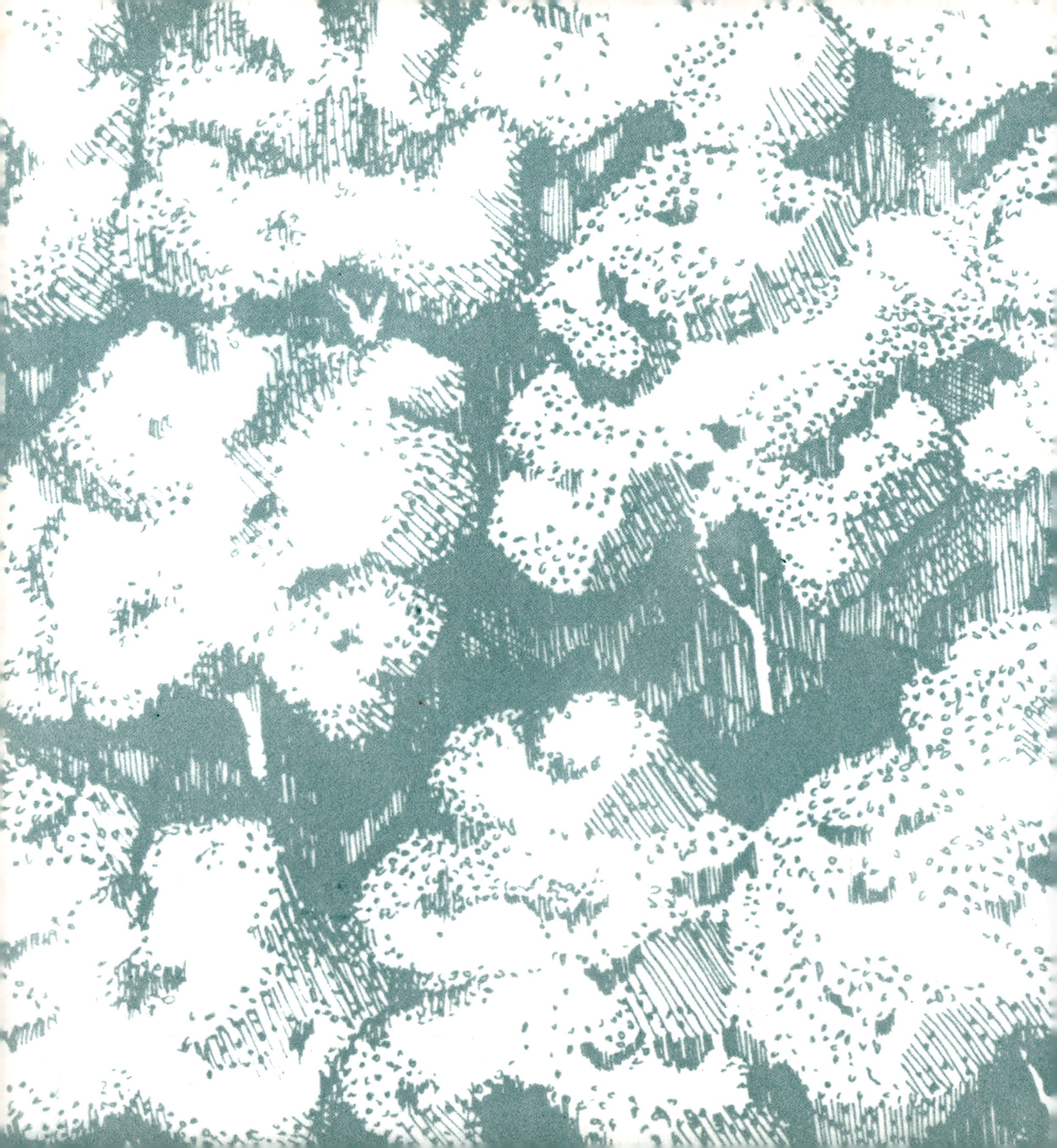